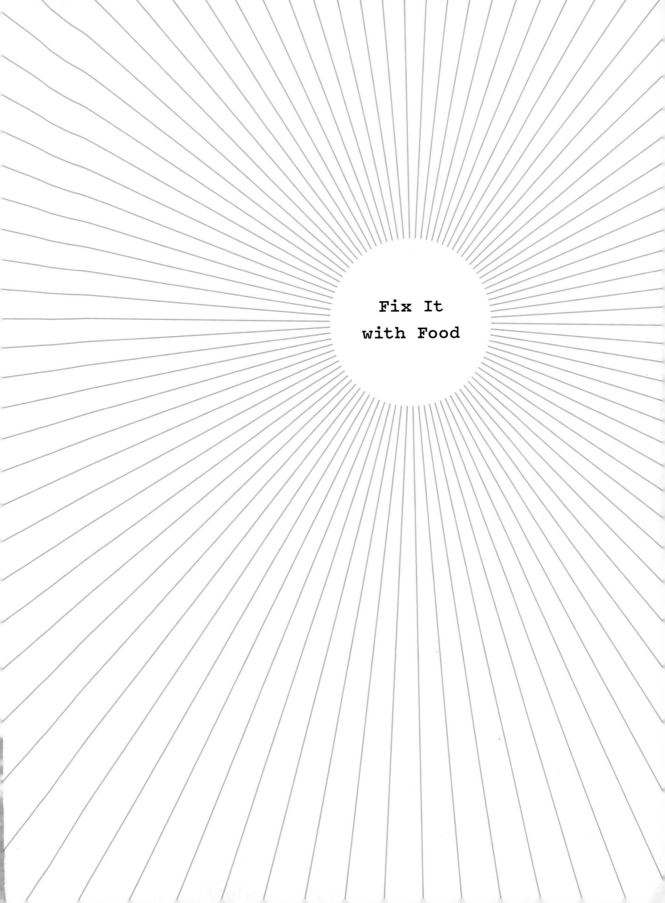

Fix It
with Food

Fix It
with

Clarkson
Potter/
Publishers

New York

More Than 125 Recipes to
Address Autoimmune Issues
and Inflammation

Food

Michael Symon
and Douglas Trattner

Photographs by Ed Anderson
Food Styling by Susan Spungen

Contents

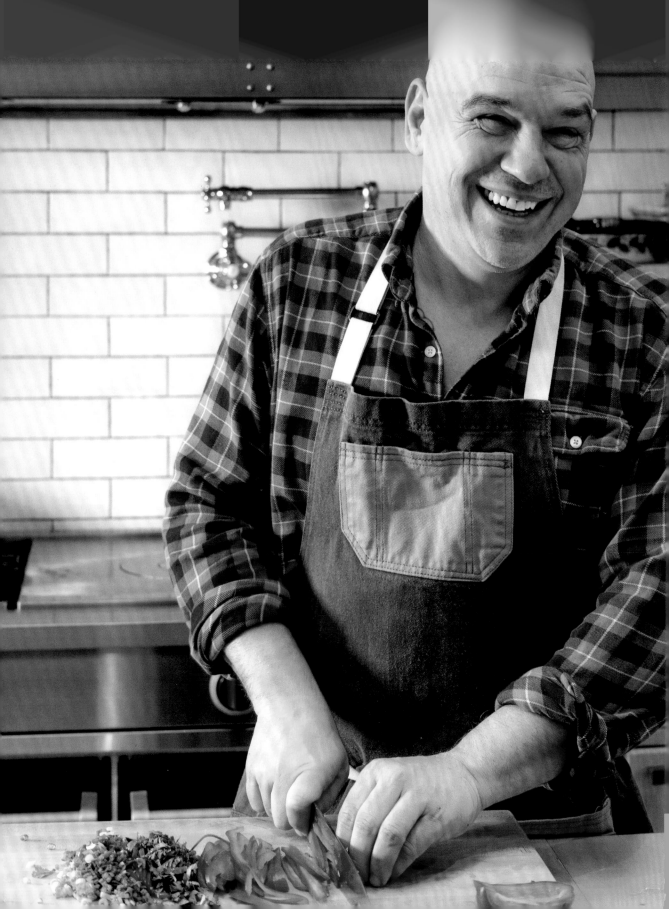

Introduction

Hi, I'm Michael Symon and I've been cooking professionally for more than thirty years. I know, I can't believe it either sometimes. One year after Liz and I opened our first restaurant, Lola in the Tremont neighborhood of Cleveland, I was named a Best New Chef by *Food & Wine* magazine. The rest, as they say, is history.

Over the years we've opened restaurants in Cleveland, Detroit, Atlantic City, and Las Vegas, where we recently debuted Mabel's BBQ at the renovated Palms Casino Resort. I've hosted or appeared on countless Food Network and Cooking Channel shows like *The Next Iron Chef,* which I won to become, well, the next Iron Chef; *Burgers, Brew & 'Que;* and *Cook Like an Iron Chef,* to name a few. For seven years, I was a cohost of *The Chew*, the popular daytime food-themed talk show.

It was my personal experiences on *The Chew,* in fact, that inspired me to write this book. I suffer from two chronic autoimmune diseases, rheumatoid arthritis and discoid lupus, an external form of the disease that affects the skin. I've always suffered a lot of joint pain—high school wrestling and thirty years on your feet in restaurant kitchens will do that to you—but it's progressively gotten worse with age. The periods between flare-ups has decreased, and the levels of pain and discomfort have increased. It was time to do something about it.

On *The Chew,* as one of my New Year's resolutions, I decided to experiment with what I now call The Reset (page 12). I used to assume that my aches and pains were simply the result of a cocktail of sports injuries, a strenuous occupation, and age (I'm not getting any younger!). Later, after I was diagnosed with rheumatoid arthritis and external lupus, I resigned myself to the fact that pain (and pain pills) would be a regular part of my life. But after I committed to doing The Reset on *The Chew,* I learned that by eating the right foods and avoiding the wrong ones, I could completely change the way I live, cook, eat, and feel.

I knew that common ingredients like sugar, flour, dairy, and red meat were often blamed for causing inflammation and the pain that comes with it, but I also recognize that everybody is different. What affects *you* negatively might not bother me. It's probably not surprising to learn that feeling good starts with eating a healthy and varied diet that's loaded with fruits, vegetables, and whole grains. Fruits and vegetables are rich in antioxidants that strengthen the immune system. Nuts and avocados are high in monounsaturated fats (the good fats), which also counter inflammation. Beans have antioxidant and anti-inflammatory qualities. And the omega-3 fatty acids found in certain types of fish like salmon, mackerel, sardines, and anchovies are great at fighting inflammation. On the other side of the coin, it is essential that you avoid chemically processed foods like cookies, chips, jarred sauces, deli meats, and many sandwich breads. Most are chock-full of added sugar, salt, and unhealthy fats, not to mention artificial colors, flavors, and preservatives. It's so important to always read the nutrition label on foods to see what ingredients are listed so that you can avoid the unhealthy ones. Alcohol also can cause inflammation for some people, especially when consuming beverages with high amounts of sugar and carbohydrates. It's up to you to decide how alcoholic beverages affect you personally, but I think at least during The Reset, it makes sense to abstain.

I wanted to dig deeper into the root causes of my inflammation to determine specifically which foods or types of food triggered painful flare-ups that could last for days. For twenty days, I followed a strict diet that avoided all foods commonly associated with inflammation (which is the source of pain) to see if what I eat—and don't eat—might affect how I feel. I was astonished to discover that by the fourth or fifth day, most of my joint pain had subsided, the skin splotches from the lupus had vanished, and I was feeling less fatigued. By the end of ten days, the improvement was dramatic. And after twenty days, I felt like a teenager again! (Okay, that might be an exaggeration.) At the end of the process I introduced an ingredient like sugar, flour, dairy, or red meat for two days to see how it affected my body. By focusing on just one potential trigger at a time, I could isolate the results and have confidence that my reactions were or were not the result of that food. I did this for each ingredient, paying close attention to my condition during each experiment. Then, I devised a food-based plan that would help me eat around my personal triggers.

Throughout my seven years on *The Chew*, I had never received as much positive feedback as I did while completing this exercise. Through Facebook, Twitter, Instagram, and email, people would reach out to share their own personal results and to request more and more recipes. It was incredibly refreshing to learn that people not only were cooking the recipes and enjoying them, but that they were also finding success in eating this way and feeling better because of them. It was then that I decided to begin this cookbook project.

This book is not intended to be used as a bible. It's a guide to help you figure out which foods trigger inflammation and cause pain and then provide delicious recipes that steer clear of those triggers. Nobody's perfect, most of all me. I know that I'm not always going to avoid detrimental foods like that bowl of ice cream on a hot summer day, or a crock of creamy mac and cheese in winter (or that second glass of bourbon!). But knowing what foods cause issues—and having at your disposal a selection of delicious recipes that avoid those triggers—puts me (and you) in control and offers the best opportunity to live pain-free while still eating well.

How to Use This Book

To ensure that you have the best possible chance at success while using this cookbook, I recommend that you take a little time up front to prepare. Read through the 10-Day Fix chapter, which I call the The Reset, and then map out what meals you intend to cook and eat. Draft a shopping list (to make life easy, see page 15 for a list we've provided that covers all of the thirty Reset recipes) and do the grocery shopping ahead of time so that you're all ready to go. Clean and prep ingredients like greens, fruits, and vegetables right when you get home from the store so that they are recipe-ready. And fill your pantry and fridge with the necessary ingredients (page 14) and healthy snacks (page 212), like those that we include in this book, to protect you from the inevitable cravings and temptations.

Drink plenty of water throughout the entire process and stick with it. Like most things worth doing, this one starts easy and gets more challenging as the days slog on and the deprivations pile up. But so, too, do the rewards, which begin to appear after just a few days and continue to multiply as you continue.

Once you discover what foods to avoid, this book makes it easy to prepare a whole host of delicious recipes without fear of reprisal. And when the inevitable happens and you've slipped, do not beat yourself up about it. Everybody backslides now and again. The best way to handle it is to treat it like a hangover: Drink plenty of water and try to avoid doing it in the future.

Top 10 Anti-inflammatory Ingredients

We've all heard the expression "Food is the best medicine." When it comes to managing inflammation, truer words have never been spoken.

By making careful decisions about what foods to eat—and which ones to avoid—I'm able to manage pain caused from inflammation without the need for pharmaceuticals. It's well established that we should strive to eat a healthy, balanced diet that includes plenty of fresh fruits and vegetables, nuts and whole grains, lean meats, and fish that is abundant in good fats. It is also known that we should attempt to avoid processed foods that are loaded with added sugar, refined grains, hydrogenated fats, stabilizers, and preservatives.

When it comes to anti-inflammatory ingredients, some foods stand out. Consider these my all-star roster of "medicinal" foods.

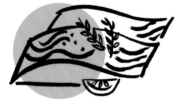

Salmon
So-called fatty fish like salmon (and mackerel, sardines, and anchovies) contain high levels of omega-3 fatty acids, which are proven to improve cardiovascular health, while fighting inflammation.

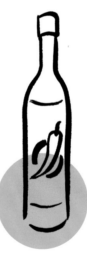

Cayenne Oil
Studies have shown that capsaicin, the active ingredient in many chile peppers, has both analgesic and anti-inflammatory properties that make it useful for both topical and edible uses.

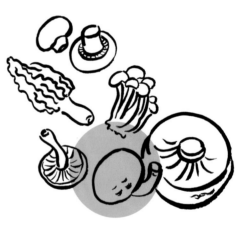

Mushrooms
Edible fungi like cremini, shiitake, and portobello mushrooms are great sources of antioxidants, vitamin D, and selenium, an essential mineral shown to help prevent inflammation.

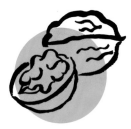

Walnuts

Nuts like walnuts (and almonds, cashews, and pecans) are rich in antioxidants, low in carbs, and high in beneficial fiber, and they possess alpha-linolenic acid, an inflammation-busting omega-3 fatty acid.

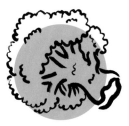

Broccoli

Brassica (also known as cruciferous) vegetables like broccoli, cauliflower, cabbage, and Brussels sprouts contain abundant amounts of disease-fighting phytochemicals like sulforaphane, which aids in reducing inflammation.

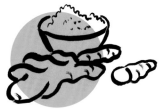

Fresh or Ground Turmeric

Curcumin, the source of turmeric's bright yellow hue, has been proven to fight inflammation. When combined with piperine-containing black pepper, those benefits are shown to greatly multiply.

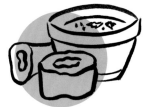

Bone Broth

Bone broth is on the receiving end of some dubious health claims. I like it not only because it tastes amazing sipped from a mug (or added to a recipe instead of beef stock), but the savory brew also contains collagen, which helps battle inflammation while improving gut health and boosting the immune system.

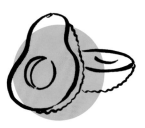

Avocado

Avocados are jam-packed with glutathione, a powerful antioxidant, and heart-healthy monounsaturated fats that are well-regarded as having anti-inflammatory qualities.

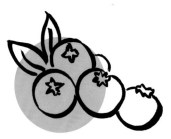

Blueberries

In addition to being loaded with antioxidants, blueberries (and strawberries and raspberries) contain colorful flavonoids that have strong anti-inflammatory qualities.

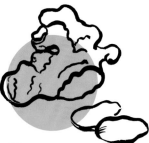

Ginger

Gingerol, the aromatic compound found in fresh ginger, helps to alleviate pain and inflammation while being a proven antioxidant.

10-Day
Fix
(aka The Reset)

Think of the 10-Day Fix like hitting the reset button. I know that it might not sound thrilling to go ten days without consuming any flour, sugar, dairy, red meat, or alcohol, but just think how good you'll feel once you know which triggers to avoid! Finally, you'll be able to better understand what to avoid to live with less pain. By eliminating all potential triggers at once, you wipe the slate clean and establish a great starting point to begin examining specific foods and their effects on your well-being. I'll admit that the first time I did this reset I struggled. For the first couple days I had headaches and felt a little lethargic, likely withdrawal from all of the hidden sugars in the peanut butter, salad dressings, and commercial breads I was consuming. Just stay strong and keep your end goal in mind. For me, by the fourth or fifth day, I was feeling great, but man was I craving many of the foods I gave up—I would have killed for a slice of pizza! At the end of the process, though, I would estimate that 95 percent of my arthritic pain was gone. To me, that's worth not giving into my cravings.

To make The Reset as easy as possible, I've included thirty delicious and nutritionally balanced recipes in this chapter—ten days of breakfast, lunch, and dinner—for you to follow like a roadmap to success. All of them are clean and free from the major potential triggers. But don't feel as if you have to stick to it like it's a set of commandments delivered from above. If you really enjoy a particular recipe, go ahead and make it again. And again. These dishes can be enjoyed in any order you want.

On the show, I did the process for twenty days, and let me tell you, it was not easy to go without all of my favorite foods for that long. Going forward, however, I learned that ten days works just as well.

Unlike the recipes in the rest of the book, most of these recipes in The Reset chapter make one serving because we assume you'll be going it alone. But if you're lucky enough to have a supportive family member, these recipes are easy to double or even triple in size to accommodate them. Others, like the Vegetable Chili (page 56), are batch-style dishes that make up to four servings so that they can be stretched across a couple meals. We've also included recipes that are designed to have leftovers that get put to use in a second dish, like the Wild Mushroom Risotto (page 55) that becomes the filling for Baked Stuffed Portobellos (page 74). By cooking certain foods ahead of time and in bigger batches, such as brown rice (page 248), quinoa (page 244), and mushroom and vegetable stocks (pages 241 and 240), you will have a jump start on a number of recipes, making your day-of meal prep more streamlined. If you want to follow the 10-Day Fix to the letter of the law, the shopping list on page 15 couldn't make it any easier.

Your Pantry

Since beginning my personal mission to manage inflammation through the foods I eat (and avoid), I've had to rethink the way I stock my pantry to make space for items like quinoa, steel-cut oats, and tamari (wheat-free soy sauce). Having ingredients like these at the ready assists me in preparing delicious recipes that avoid triggers like flour, sugar, dairy, and meat with relative ease.

Pantry staples like spices, nuts, seeds, and oils do not live forever. While most spices will last longer than one year (depending on storage), I elect to start fresh every year to ensure that my spices are fresh, aromatic, and potent. I prefer to buy spices in whole form whenever possible (whole spices last longer than ground spices) and toast, crush, and/or grind them as needed. A freshly toasted and ground spice is superior to one that was ground many moons ago. The natural oils in nuts and seeds can go rancid in as little as a few months when improperly stored. Always opt for an airtight container stashed in a dark space. To up that shelf life from six months to one year, store the airtight container in the fridge. And to squeeze out two years or more from nuts and seeds, pop the container in the freezer.

Throughout this book you'll see the option to substitute "good-quality canned or boxed broth" for recipe ingredients like Mushroom Stock (page 241) and Vegetable Stock (page 240). While homemade stock tastes better, is usually more nutritious, and costs a fraction of the price (especially when using trimmings and leftovers) compared to most commercial brands, I understand that making them from scratch is not always practical, so of course it's fine to use store-bought. Look for low-sodium versions of organic brands and read the nutrition label so you can avoid additives like MSG, yeast extract, and the anything-but-natural "natural flavors."

When it comes to bone broth, however, commercial beef stocks and broths are not in the same league as real bone broth, which is made by slowly simmering meaty beef bones for hours on end to extract all the amazing flavors and beneficial vitamins, minerals, and collagen (check out page 237 for my Beef Bone Broth recipe). I always cook up a big batch and freeze it in small portions so I can grab a pint or two as I need it.

Pantry

Oils
Extra-virgin olive oil
Coconut oil
Grapeseed oil

Grains, Oats, Beans
Steel-cut oats
Brown rice
Arborio rice
Quinoa
Canned chickpeas
Canned black beans

Vinegars and Seasonings
Red wine vinegar
Balsamic vinegar
White distilled vinegar
Sherry vinegar
Apple cider vinegar
Tamari (wheat-free soy sauce)
Dijon mustard

Spices
Kosher salt
Black peppercorns
Ground cinnamon
Ground turmeric
Sweet paprika
Smoked paprika
Whole coriander
Ground coriander
Ground cumin
Curry powder
Garlic powder
Cayenne

10-Day Reset Shopping List

To make preparing for The Reset as effortless as possible, I assembled a detailed shopping list of all the foods. Bring this list to the grocery store (or snap a photo of it on your phone), and you'll be all set for your 10-day journey. Herbs and vegetables are freshest and healthiest used within 5 days, so take a close look at the recipes that you'll be making over the first few days, and check the ingredients against the contents of your fridge before shopping. On Day 4 or 5 of The Reset, assess your fridge, check your shopping list, and replenish what's running low or needs to be purchased to get you through Day 10.

Legumes, Nuts, and Seeds

2 cups dried black-eyed peas
2 tablespoons dry-roasted salted peanuts
1 cup walnut halves
¼ cup slivered almonds
1 cup raw cashews
6 tablespoons pine nuts
¾ cup pepitas
1 tablespoon chia seeds

Fresh Herbs

1 bunch flat-leaf parsley
6 scallions
Small bunch thyme
Small bunch rosemary
1 bunch cilantro
Small bunch oregano
6 bay leaves

Fruit

6 lemons
4 limes
2 navel oranges
2 Granny Smith apples
2 avocados
1½ cups strawberries
1 cup chopped pineapple
1 banana
½ cup blueberries

Vegetables

Leafy Greens

6 cups baby spinach
7 cups Lacinato kale leaves
2 cups collard green leaves
5 cups Swiss chard leaves
1 small head Bibb lettuce
1 small endive
1 cup arugula

Hardy Vegetables

12 medium carrots
12 ribs celery
6 medium yellow onions
6 leeks
4 medium sweet potatoes
4 radishes
4 heads garlic
2 cups broccoli florets
2 small heads cauliflower
2 cups Brussels sprouts
1 zucchini
1 medium Yukon Gold potato
1 small butternut squash
1 large hand ginger

Tender/Perishable Vegetables

5 jalapeños
3 red bell peppers
2 cups green beans
2 medium eggplants
2 bulbs fennel
1 English cucumber
1 cup grape tomatoes
1 large bunch asparagus
1 green bell pepper

Mushrooms

5 cups wild mushrooms
4 medium portobellos
4 cups cremini mushrooms

Miscellaneous

2 dozen large eggs
2 (15-ounce) cans full-fat coconut milk
2 (15-ounce) cans crushed San Marzano tomatoes
1 cup unsweetened almond milk
¼ cup nutritional yeast
2 ounces dried porcini mushrooms
2 tablespoons unsweetened cocoa powder
2 tablespoons dried cherries
1 tablespoon golden raisins

10-Day Fix Menus

I know from personal experience how intimidating it can be to commit to something like the 10-Day Reset. I made a similar pledge in front of millions of viewers on live television! The good news is that every single one of these recipes is delicious and nutritious, meaning that you will never feel cheated, hungry, or (hopefully!) cranky. Keep your eye on the prize and know that you will begin to feel amazing in a couple days and, by the end, be well on your way to managing your own inflammation and pain through cooking and food. (And a heads-up—you'll need to have Oregano Oil, page 244; Dairy-Free Parmesan, page 241; and Cayenne Oil, page 246, on hand for The Reset, so make these pantry items before kicking off the 10-Day Reset to keep your day-to-day cooking efficient and streamlined.)

Day 1

Rolled Spinach Omelet
page 18

Kale Salad with Radishes,
Zucchini, and Tomatoes
page 21

Roasted Broccoli with
Cauliflower Puree
page 22

Day 2

Oatmeal with Blueberries,
Walnuts, and Cinnamon
page 24

Quinoa and Egg Salad with
Chickpeas and Asparagus
page 27

Sweet Potato Pancakes
with Wilted Greens
page 28

Day 3

Morning Sunrise Smoothie
page 30

Green Bean and Walnut Salad
with a Poached Egg
page 33

Grilled Portobellos with
Arugula and Olive Oil
Mashed Potatoes
page 34

Day 4

Baked Eggs over Greens
page 36

Crispy Stir-Fried Brown
Rice with Wild Mushrooms
page 39

Stuffed Butternut
Squash page 40

Day 5

Green Machine Smoothie
page 42

Baked Sweet Potato
with Black-Eyed Pea Stew
page 43

Quinoa Black Bean Burger
with Cucumber Salad
page 45

Day 6

Baked Eggs in Avocado
with Peppers page 46

Warm Spinach and Mushroom
Salad with Pine Nuts
page 48

Stuffed Peppers with
Black-Eyed Peas and
Quinoa page 51

Day 7

Sweet Potato and Kale
Hash with Fried Eggs
page 52

Wild Mushroom Risotto
page 55

Vegetable Chili
page 56

Day 8

Avocado and Tomato Egg
Scramble page 58

Sweet Potato and Coconut
Stew page 61

Grilled Spiced Cauliflower
Steaks with Jeweled Rice
page 62

Day 9

Oatmeal with Coconut
Cream, Strawberries, and
Toasted Almonds page 64

Bibb Salad with Apples,
Squash, and Walnuts
page 67

Veggie Stir-Fry
over Brown Rice
page 68

Day 10

Almond, Berry, and Chia
Smoothie with Spinach
page 70

Brussels Sprouts, Apple,
and Brown Rice Salad
page 73

Baked Stuffed
Portobellos
page 74

Day 1

We kick-start The Reset with a day jam-packed with leafy greens, brassicas, and vegetables. For breakfast is an omelet that comes together in minutes, but powers you all the way to lunch thanks to nutrient-dense spinach. A classic vinaigrette transforms thin-sliced kale and crunchy veggies into a light but satisfying lunch that can be bundled up to go. Dinner stars blistered broccoli and crunchy nuts served on a creamy bed of cauliflower puree. So good!

Rolled Spinach Omelet

Day 1
Breakfast

Serves 1

2 tablespoons **extra-virgin olive oil**

1 cup **spinach leaves**

Kosher salt and freshly ground black pepper

3 large **eggs**, beaten

½ teaspoon **Oregano Oil** (page 244)

1. Set a medium nonstick skillet over medium heat. Add the olive oil and heat to shimmering, then add the spinach. Season with a pinch of salt and a twist of black pepper. Cook, stirring occasionally, until the spinach begins to wilt, about 30 seconds.

2. Add the eggs and cook, occasionally using a silicone spatula to gently push the cooked eggs in from the outer edge. Tilt the pan so that the liquid eggs fill the now-vacant spaces. When the eggs are almost set throughout, season them with another pinch of salt and twist of pepper and drizzle with oregano oil.

3. To serve, tilt the skillet and gently roll the omelet out onto a plate.

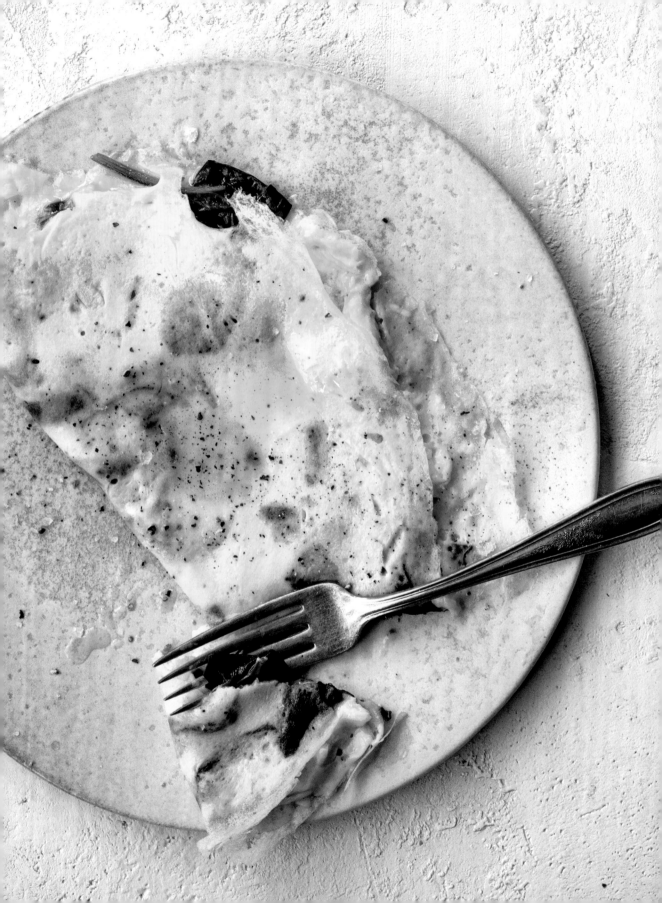

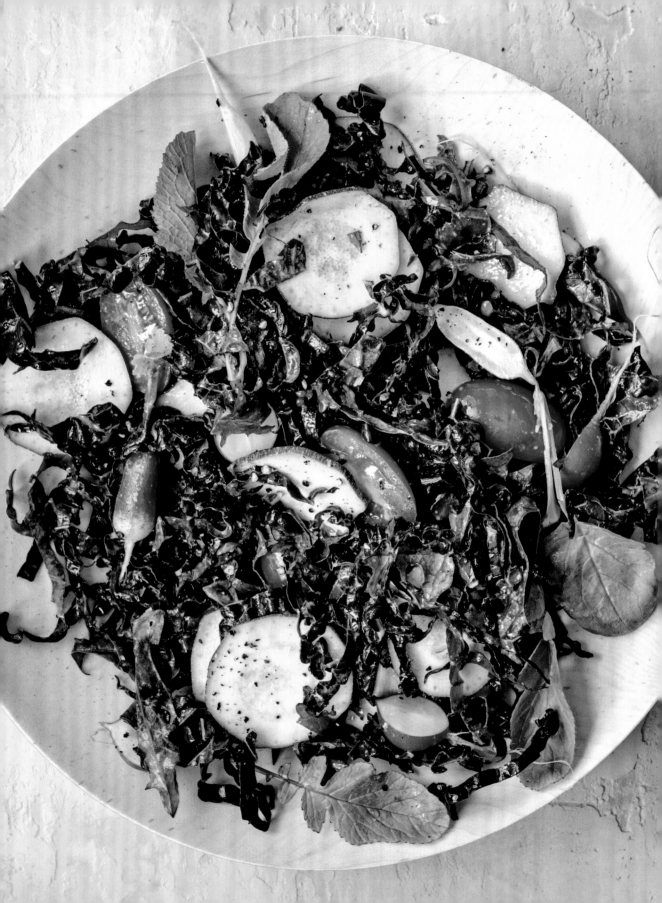

Kale Salad

with Radishes, Zucchini, and Tomatoes

Serves 1

6 **kale leaves and tender stems**, thinly sliced (about 3 cups)

2 tablespoons **extra-virgin olive oil**

1 tablespoon **red wine vinegar**

1 teaspoon **Dijon mustard**

Kosher salt and freshly ground black pepper

4 **radishes**, quartered (or halved if small)

½ **zucchini**, thinly sliced (about ½ cup)

½ cup **grape tomatoes**, halved

1. In a large bowl, vigorously massage the kale leaves with both hands until the kale darkens and breaks down, about 3 minutes. Set aside.

2. In another large bowl, whisk together the olive oil, vinegar, and mustard. Season with a pinch of salt and a twist of black pepper. Add the kale, radishes, zucchini, and tomatoes. Season with more salt and pepper and toss together.

Roasted Broccoli

with Cauliflower Puree

Day 1
Dinner

Serves 2

2 cups **broccoli florets**

7 tablespoons **extra-virgin olive oil**

Kosher salt and freshly ground black pepper

3 cups roughly chopped **cauliflower** (about ½ head)

2 tablespoons **Dairy-Free Parmesan** (page 241), plus more for serving

2 tablespoons **salted roasted peanuts**

Juice of ½ small **lime**

2 tablespoons finely chopped **fresh flat-leaf parsley**

1 tablespoon **Cayenne Oil** (page 246)

1. Preheat the oven to 425°F. Line a sheet pan with parchment paper.

2. Arrange the broccoli on the lined pan, making sure to leave some space between the florets. Drizzle with 2 tablespoons of the olive oil, season with a few pinches of salt and twists of black pepper, and roast until the broccoli is nicely charred and cooked through, about 15 minutes.

3. Meanwhile, set a large heavy-bottomed skillet over medium-high heat. Add 3 tablespoons of the olive oil and heat to shimmering, then add the cauliflower and a pinch of salt. Cook until the cauliflower begins to soften and brown, about 5 minutes. Add 1 cup water and deglaze the pan, scraping with a wooden spoon to get up the browned bits from the bottom of the pan. Continue cooking, uncovered, until most of the liquid has evaporated and the cauliflower is fully cooked, about 8 minutes.

4. Transfer the cauliflower to a blender or food processor. Add the remaining 2 tablespoons olive oil and the Dairy-Free Parmesan and puree until very smooth. Taste and add more salt and pepper if needed.

5. In a large bowl, combine the roasted broccoli, peanuts, lime juice, parsley, and cayenne oil and toss together. Taste and add salt and pepper if needed.

6. Serve the roasted broccoli mixture on top of the cauliflower puree. Garnish with more Dairy-Free Parmesan, if desired.

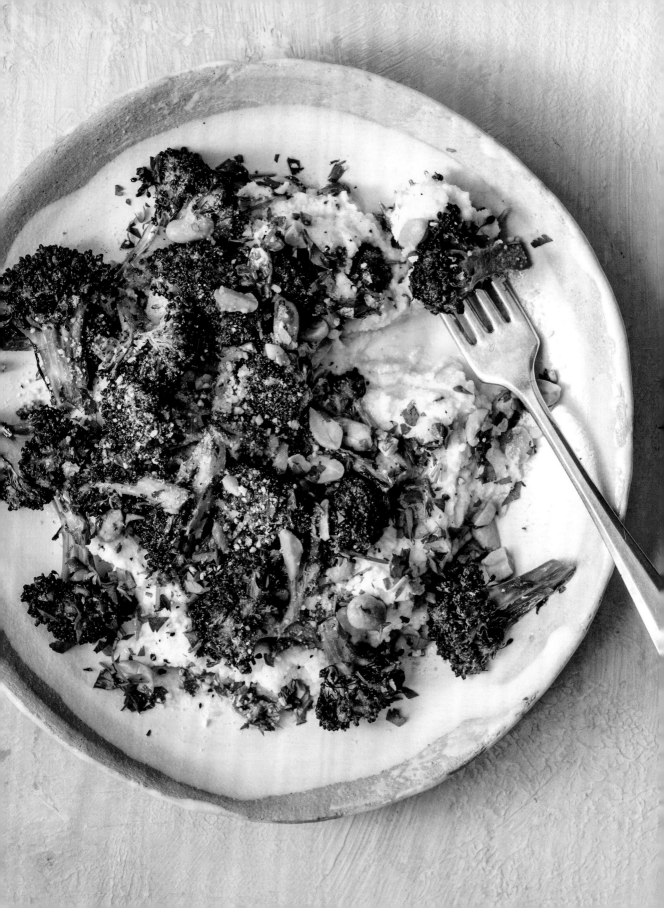

Day 2

I've been trying to add more healthy nuts and whole grains into my diet, and one of the easiest ways to do that is by topping a bowl of comforting oatmeal with freshly roasted walnuts. The salad for lunch is light, nutty, and fresh, but it's also filling thanks to the protein-packed, hard-cooked egg. Crispy pan-fried sweet potato pancakes set against savory sautéed greens is the weekday dinner that you didn't know was missing from your repertoire.

Oatmeal
with Blueberries, Walnuts, and Cinnamon

Day 2
Breakfast

Serves 1

¼ cup **walnut halves**

1 tablespoon **coconut oil**

⅓ cup **steel-cut oats**

½ cup **unsweetened full-fat coconut milk**

Kosher salt

½ cup **blueberries**

½ teaspoon **ground cinnamon**

1. Preheat the oven to 350°F.

2. Arrange the walnuts on a sheet pan and cook until lightly toasted, about 8 minutes. Transfer to a cutting board and once they are cool enough to handle, roughly chop and set aside.

3. Set a medium saucepan over medium heat. Add the coconut oil and the oats and cook, stirring occasionally, until fragrant, about 1 minute. Add the coconut milk, ¾ cup water, and a pinch of salt. Bring to a simmer and cook, stirring occasionally, until the oats are tender, about 45 minutes.

4. Remove the oats from the heat and serve topped with blueberries, cinnamon, and walnuts.

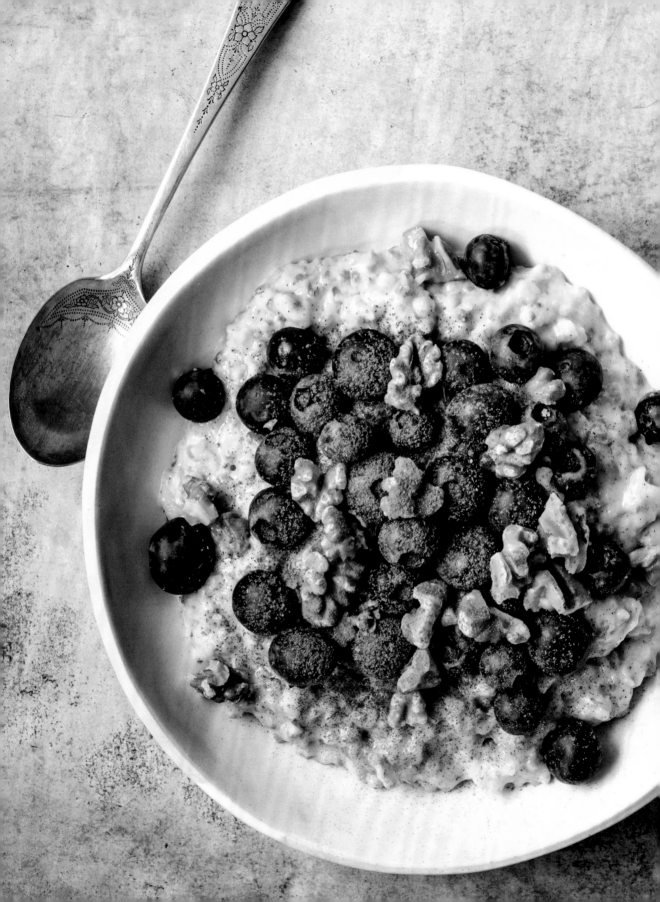

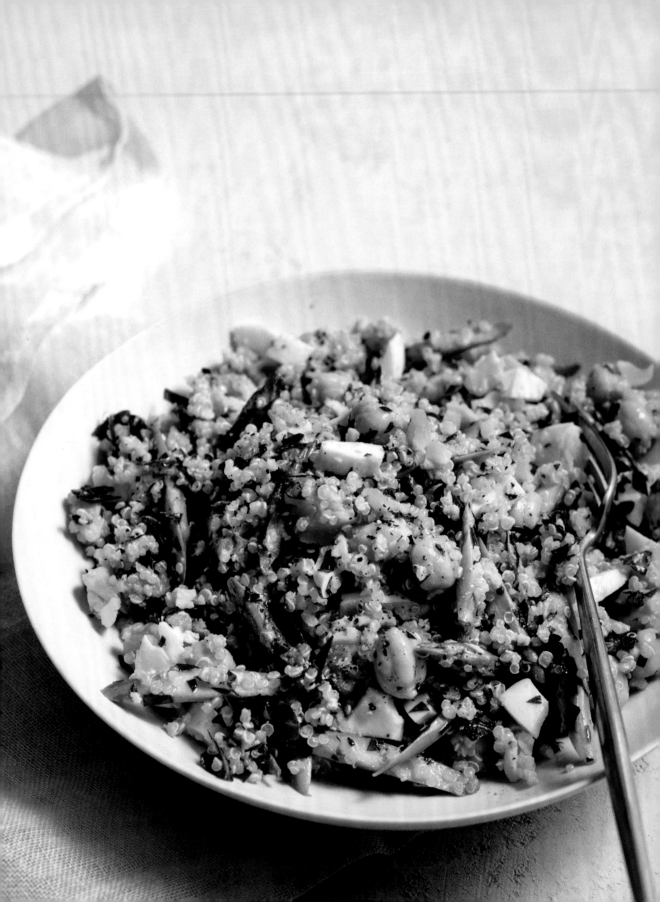

Quinoa and Egg Salad

with Chickpeas and Asparagus

Serves 1

1 large **egg**

3 tablespoons **Oregano Oil** (page 244)

1 tablespoon **red wine vinegar**

1 tablespoon **fresh lemon juice**

1 teaspoon **Dijon mustard**

Kosher salt and freshly ground black pepper

1 cup **cooked Quinoa** (page 244)

½ cup **cooked chickpeas**, drained and rinsed if using canned

½ cup thinly sliced **asparagus**

2 tablespoons roughly chopped **fresh flat-leaf parsley**

1. Place the egg in a small saucepan, cover with cold water by 1 inch, and bring to a boil over high heat. Remove from the heat, cover the pan, and set aside for 10 minutes. Drain and chill the egg in cold water for 1 minute. When the egg is cool, peel and roughly chop.

2. Meanwhile, in a medium bowl, whisk together the oregano oil, vinegar, lemon juice, and mustard. Season with a pinch of salt and a twist of black pepper.

3. Add the chopped egg, quinoa, chickpeas, asparagus, and parsley to the dressing and toss together.

Sweet Potato Pancakes

with Wilted Greens

Serves 1

1 **sweet potato**, peeled and grated on the large holes of a box grater

1 **scallion**, finely sliced

¼ teaspoon **ground turmeric**

¼ teaspoon **paprika**

1 large **egg**, beaten

Kosher salt and freshly ground black pepper

3 tablespoons **extra-virgin olive oil**

4 **collard green leaves**, tough stems removed, leaves thinly sliced (about 2 cups)

1. In a large bowl, combine the sweet potato, scallion, turmeric, paprika, and egg. Season with a pinch of salt and a twist of black pepper and toss together. Form the mixture into 3 equal-size patties and set aside.

2. Set a large skillet over medium-high heat. Add 2 tablespoons of the olive oil and heat to shimmering, then add the patties, flattening them slightly with a spatula. Cook until crisp and golden brown on both sides, about 3 minutes per side. Transfer to a plate and loosely tent with foil to keep warm.

3. To the same skillet, add the remaining 1 tablespoon olive oil, the collards, and a pinch of salt. Cook, stirring occasionally, until the greens are wilted, about 5 minutes.

4. Serve the cooked greens with the sweet potato pancakes.

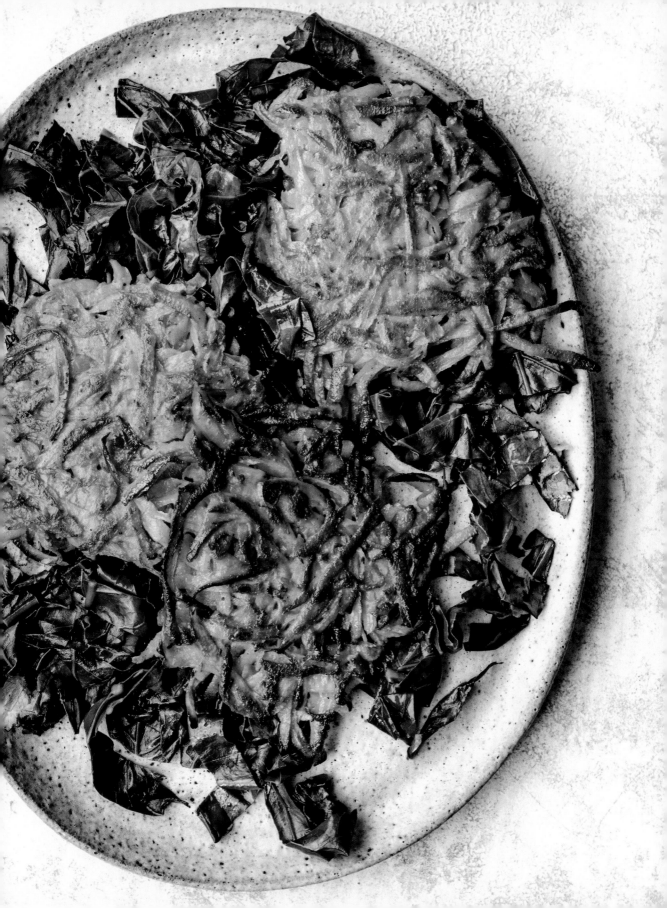

Day 3

Fruit and vegetable smoothies are popular breakfast foods for good reason: They are fast, easy, nutritious, delicious, and portable! This one is like a liquid sunset in a glass. At lunch, a delicately poached egg turns a green bean salad into a silky indulgence thanks to the runny yolk, which fortifies the dressing. You won't miss red meat for dinner when there are meaty grilled portobellos around. These are served atop comforting mashed potatoes.

Morning Sunrise Smoothie

Day 3
Breakfast

Makes 1 smoothie

2 medium **carrots**, diced

1 cup fresh or frozen **pineapple chunks**

2-inch piece **fresh ginger**, peeled and roughly chopped

1 tablespoon **coconut oil**

1 teaspoon **ground turmeric**

Juice of 1 lemon

1 cup **water**

In a blender, combine all of the ingredients and process until smooth.

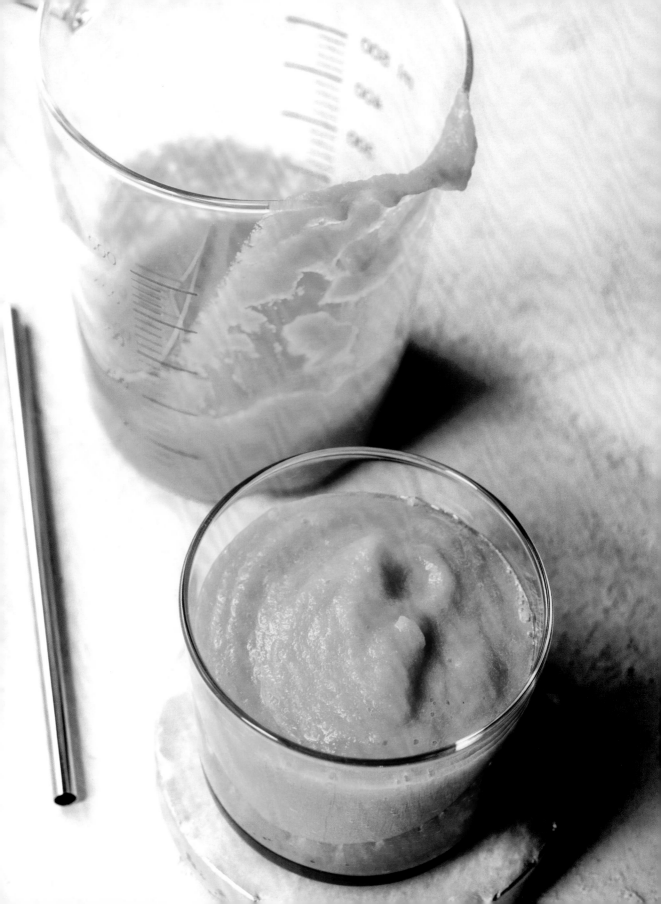

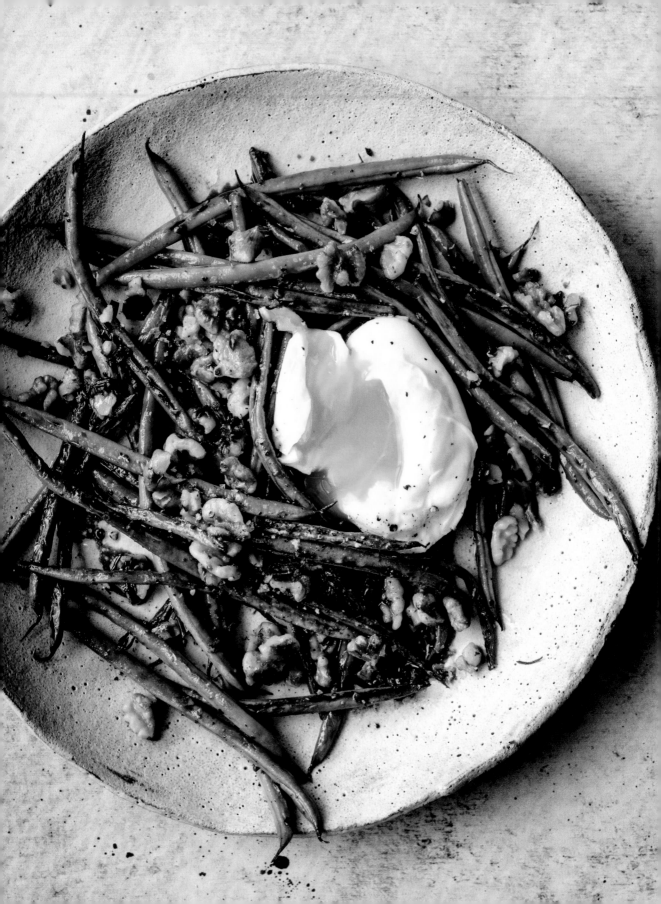

Green Bean and Walnut Salad

with a Poached Egg

Serves 1

2 tablespoons **balsamic vinegar**

1 teaspoon **Dijon mustard**

2 tablespoons **extra-virgin olive oil**

2 cups **green beans**, ends trimmed

**Kosher salt and freshly ground
   black pepper**

⅓ cup roughly **chopped walnuts**

1 teaspoon **fresh thyme leaves**

2 tablespoons **distilled white vinegar**

1 large **egg**

1. In a small bowl, whisk together the balsamic vinegar and mustard. Set aside.

2. Set a large skillet over medium heat. Add the oil and heat it to shimmering, then add the green beans. Shake the pan so the beans are in an even layer, season with a pinch of salt and a twist of black pepper, and cook, without stirring, until the beans begin to char and soften, about 6 minutes. Add the walnuts and thyme, stir, and continue cooking until the walnuts are toasted and aromatic, about 1 minute. Remove from the heat, add the vinaigrette, and toss together.

3. Meanwhile, in a medium saucepan, combine 4 cups water and the white vinegar and bring to a strong simmer over medium-high heat. Crack the egg into its own little bowl. With a spoon, create a large (but gentle) whirlpool in the simmering water by stirring in one direction around the perimeter of the pan. Gently lower the egg into the center of the pan and stop stirring. Poach, untouched, until the egg is set enough to be lifted out of the water without breaking but the yolk is still runny, about 3 minutes. Gently lift the egg out of the water with a slotted spoon.

4. Add the green bean salad to a bowl and serve the egg on top of the green beans. Season with salt and pepper.

Grilled Portobellos

with Arugula and
Olive Oil Mashed
Potatoes

Day 3
Dinner

Serves 1

4 tablespoons **extra-virgin olive oil**

Juice of 1 lemon

1 **garlic clove**, minced

2 teaspoons finely chopped **fresh rosemary**

Kosher salt and freshly ground black pepper

2 medium **portobello mushrooms**, stems and gills removed

1 medium **Yukon Gold potato**, peeled and cut into 1-inch pieces

1 cup **fresh arugula**

1. In a large bowl, whisk together 2 tablespoons of the olive oil, the lemon juice, garlic, and rosemary. Season with a pinch of salt and a twist of black pepper. Add the mushroom caps, toss to coat, and set aside to marinate for 30 minutes.

2. Meanwhile, place the potatoes in a medium saucepan, cover with cold water by a few inches, add a large pinch of salt, and bring to a boil over high heat. Cook at a gentle boil until easily pierced by a fork, about 20 minutes. Drain the potatoes, reserving ¼ cup of the cooking water. Return the potatoes to the pan, add the remaining 2 tablespoons olive oil, and mash until creamy and smooth. Use the reserved cooking water to achieve the desired creamy consistency. Season with black pepper and keep warm.

3. Preheat a grill or grill pan to medium-high heat. Reserving the marinade, scoop out the mushroom caps and transfer to the grill. Cook until soft and charred on both sides, about 3 minutes per side. Transfer to a cutting board and slice in ½-inch strips.

4. Meanwhile, add the arugula to the reserved mushroom marinade and toss to coat.

5. Mound the potato puree on a plate and arrange the mushroom slices over the puree. Top with arugula salad and serve.

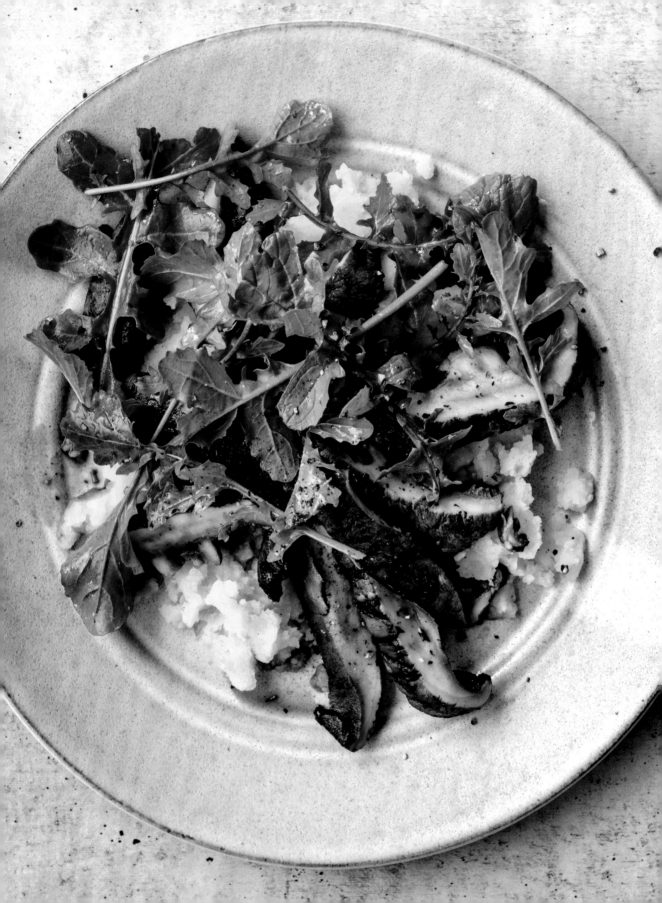

Day 4

Eggs nestled in braised greens and baked in the oven is a stress-free version of poached eggs; you get the benefit of egg whites and runny yolks, but without all the fuss. Lunch is mushroom and brown rice stir-fry loaded with rich umami flavor that I think works great hot from the skillet or at room temperature. Savory, sweet butternut squash makes the perfect base for an herby sautéed Swiss chard and quinoa medley. (A note: Don't forget to soak the black-eyed peas for tomorrow's lunch!)

Baked Eggs over Greens

Serves 1

Day 4
Breakfast

1 tablespoon **extra-virgin olive oil**

2 **scallions**, finely sliced

1 **garlic clove**, minced

Kosher salt and freshly ground black pepper

6 **Swiss chard leaves**, stemmed and sliced (about 2 cups)

1 teaspoon **fresh thyme leaves**

2 large **eggs**

1. Preheat the oven to 375°F.

2. Set a medium ovenproof skillet over medium heat. Add the olive oil and heat to shimmering, then add the scallions, garlic, and a pinch of salt. Cook until the scallions begin to soften, about 2 minutes. Add the Swiss chard and thyme and cook until the greens are wilted, about 3 minutes. Season with another pinch of salt and a twist of black pepper.

3. Make 2 shallow depressions in the vegetable mixture and carefully crack an egg into each one. Transfer the skillet to the oven and bake until the egg whites are set but the yolks are still runny, about 8 minutes (or 10 if you like your yolks more set).

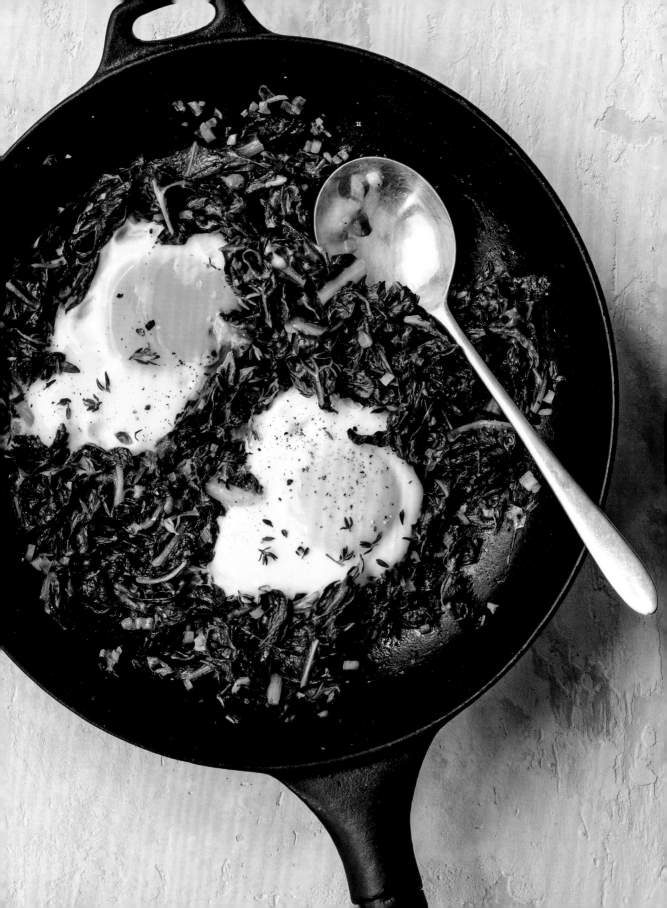

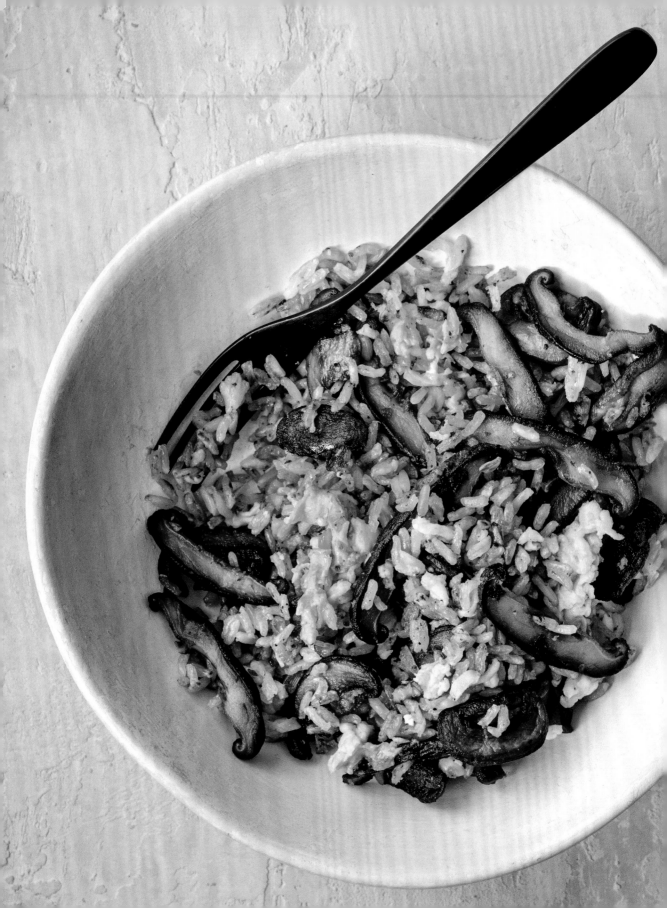

Crispy Stir-Fried Brown Rice

with Wild Mushrooms

Serves 1

3 tablespoons **extra-virgin olive oil**

2 cups sliced mixed **wild mushrooms** (such as shiitake, cremini, oyster), tough stems removed

Kosher salt and freshly ground black pepper

1 cup cooked **Brown Rice** (page 248)

2 teaspoons grated **fresh ginger**

1 **garlic clove**, minced

1 large **egg**, beaten

1 teaspoon **tamari** (wheat-free soy sauce)

1. Set a large nonstick skillet over medium-high heat. Add the oil and heat to shimmering, then add the mushrooms. Cook, without stirring, until they begin to brown and crisp on one side, about 3 minutes. Shake the pan to turn the mushrooms, season with a pinch of salt and a twist of black pepper, and add the cooked rice, ginger, and garlic, but don't stir. When the second sides of the mushrooms are browned and crispy, continue cooking, stirring occasionally, for 3 minutes.

2. Add the egg and cook, stirring occasionally, until the egg is set, about 1 minute. Remove from the heat, stir in the tamari, and serve.

10-Day Fix

Stuffed Butternut Squash

Day 4
Dinner

Serves 1

2 tablespoons **pine nuts**

½ small **butternut squash**, seeded (save the other ½ squash for Bibb Salad with Apples, Squash, and Walnuts, page 67)

3 tablespoons **extra-virgin olive oil**, plus more for drizzling

Kosher salt and freshly ground black pepper

½ cup finely diced **yellow onion**

1 **garlic clove**, minced

½ cup **cooked Quinoa** (page 244)

6 **Swiss chard leaves**, stemmed and sliced (about 3 cups)

2 tablespoons finely chopped **fresh flat-leaf parsley**

1. Preheat the oven to 350°F.

2. Place the pine nuts on a sheet pan and cook until lightly toasted, about 8 minutes. Set aside.

3. Increase the oven temperature to 425°F. Line a sheet pan with foil.

4. Place the squash half cut-side up on the lined sheet pan. Coat the exposed flesh with 1 tablespoon of the olive oil, season with salt and pepper, and roast until golden brown, about 45 minutes. Flip and continue cooking until the squash is easily pierced with a knife, about 20 minutes more.

5. Meanwhile, set a large skillet over medium heat. Add the remaining 2 tablespoons olive oil and heat to shimmering, then add the onion, garlic, and a pinch of salt. Cook until the onion softens, about 2 minutes. Add the cooked quinoa and Swiss chard and cook, stirring occasionally, until the greens are wilted, about 3 minutes. Season with another pinch of salt and a twist of black pepper. Remove from the heat and stir in the pine nuts and parsley.

6. Mound the greens onto the squash, drizzle with olive oil, and serve.

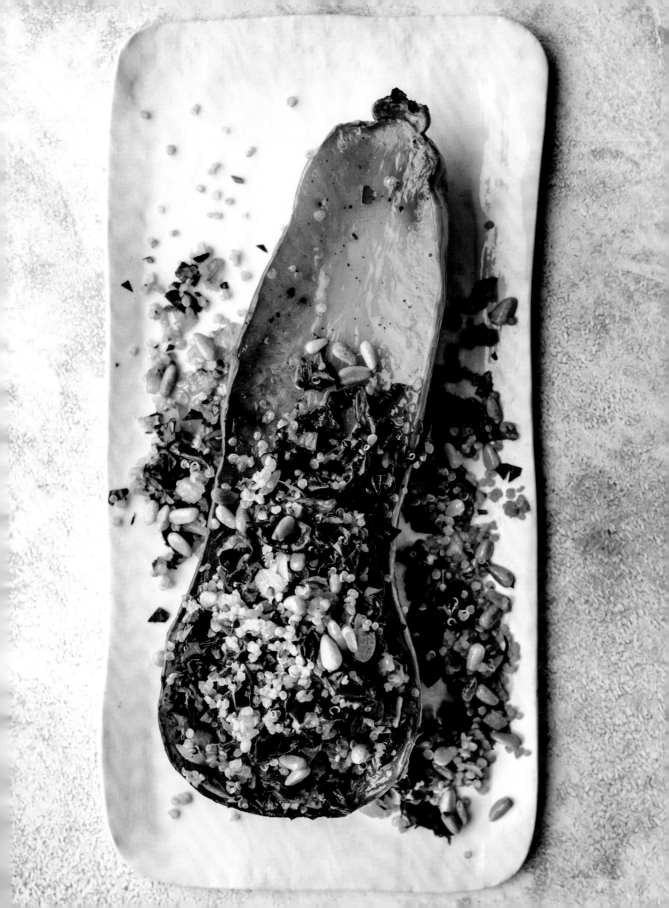

Day 5

The Green Machine Smoothie (below) might not win any awards for appearance, but it's packed with protein and makes for a refreshing eye-opener thanks to the apple, orange, lemon, and ginger. Soul food in the form of a black-eyed pea stew with warm spices makes an appearance at lunch atop a luscious sweet potato. It took serious recipe testing to perfect my quinoa and black bean burgers, but I couldn't be happier with the results. Served with a bright and crunchy cucumber salad, they make a great meal any day of the week—even after you're done with The Reset!

Green Machine Smoothie

Day 5
Breakfast

Makes 1 smoothie

4 **kale leaves with stems**, chopped (about 2 cups)

¼ medium **cucumber**, diced

2 **celery ribs**, diced

½ **Granny Smith apple**, unpeeled, cored, and roughly chopped

1 **orange**, peeled and roughly chopped

Juice of 1 lemon

2-inch piece ginger, peeled and roughly chopped

1 cup **water**

In a blender, combine all of the ingredients and process until smooth.

Baked Sweet Potato

with Black-Eyed Pea Stew

Day 5
Lunch

Serves 1 (the stew makes enough for this recipe plus the Stuffed Peppers with Black-Eyed Peas and Quinoa, page 51)

1 cup **dried black-eyed peas**, soaked overnight in cold water

1 medium **sweet potato**

2 tablespoons **extra-virgin olive oil**

1 small **yellow onion**, cut into ¼-inch dice

2 **garlic cloves**, minced

1 **jalapeño**, seeded and finely chopped

Kosher salt and freshly ground black pepper

1 **green bell pepper**, cut into ¼-inch dice

1 teaspoon **ground coriander**

½ teaspoon **ground cumin**

½ teaspoon **paprika**

1 (14.5- to 15-ounce) can **crushed San Marzano tomatoes**

2 cups **Vegetable Stock**, homemade (page 240) or good-quality canned or boxed

1 tablespoon **sherry vinegar**

1. Drain and rinse the black-eyed peas and set aside.

2. Preheat the oven to 400°F. Line a sheet pan with foil.

3. Pierce the sweet potato with a fork or paring knife a few times and roast on the lined pan until it is easily pierced with a knife, about 45 minutes.

4. Meanwhile, set a medium saucepan over medium-high heat. Add the olive oil and heat to shimmering, then add the onion, garlic, jalapeño, and a pinch of salt. Cook until the vegetables soften, about 3 minutes. Add the bell pepper, coriander, cumin, and paprika and cook, stirring occasionally, until the vegetables soften, about 2 minutes. Add the black-eyed peas, tomatoes, and stock and bring to a simmer. Cook, partially covered, until the black-eyed peas are tender, about 1 hour. Season with another pinch of salt and a twist of black pepper. Remove from the heat and stir in the vinegar. Taste and add salt and pepper, if needed. (Set aside some of the stew to serve over the sweet potatoes and refrigerate the remainder in an airtight container to use in Stuffed Peppers with Black-Eyed Peas and Quinoa on page 51.)

5. Slice the sweet potato down the middle to open, top with stew, and serve.

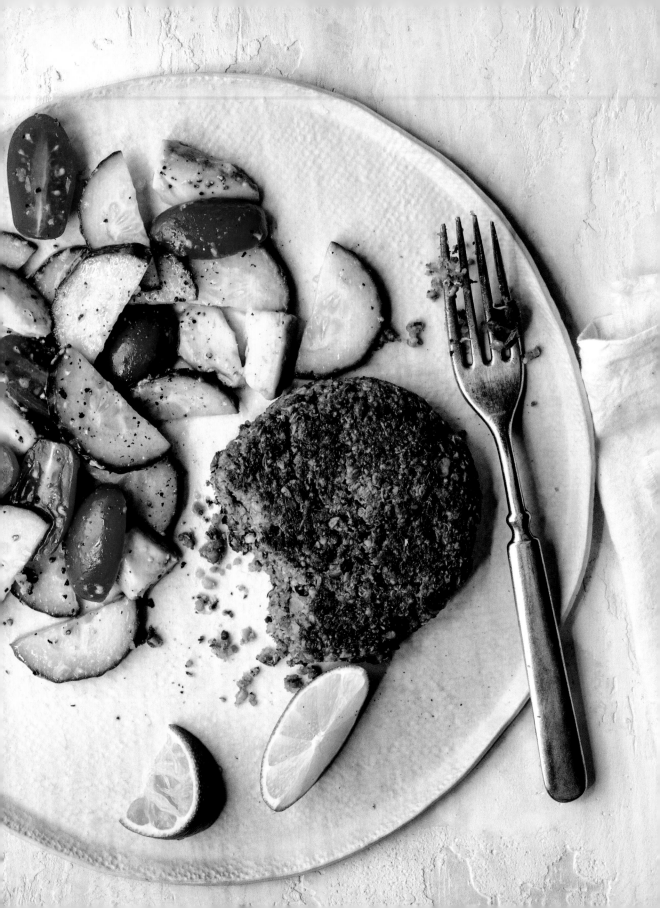

Quinoa Black Bean Burger

with Cucumber Salad

Makes 8 burgers

½ cup **roasted pumpkin seeds** (pepitas)

1 (15-ounce) can **black beans**, drained and rinsed

3½ tablespoons **extra-virgin olive oil**

2 cups **cooked Quinoa** (page 244)

1 large **egg**, beaten

2 **scallions**, finely sliced

1 teaspoon **smoked paprika**

¾ cup **Dairy-Free Parmesan** (page 241)

Kosher salt and freshly ground black pepper

½ **avocado**, diced

¼ cup halved **grape tomatoes**

¼ cup diced **cucumber**

Juice of ½ lime

1. In a food processor, pulse the pumpkin seeds until they resemble coarse bread crumbs, about 5 times. Remove and set aside.

2. Add the black beans to the food processor and pulse until they resemble a coarse mash, about 5 times. Add 2 tablespoons of the olive oil and ½ cup of the cooked quinoa and process to a sticky paste, about 1 minute.

3. Transfer the black beans to a large bowl and stir in the pumpkin seeds, the remaining 1½ cups quinoa, the egg, scallions, paprika, Dairy-Free Parmesan, ½ teaspoon salt, and ½ teaspoon black pepper. Form the mixture into 8 equal-size patties. Refrigerate them for 3 days or freeze up to 1 month.

4. Season both sides of a patty with salt and pepper. Set a medium heavy-bottomed skillet over medium heat. Add ½ tablespoon of the olive oil to the pan and heat to shimmering, then add the patty. Cook until crisp and browned on both sides, about 2 minutes per side.

5. Meanwhile, in a medium bowl, combine the avocado, tomatoes, cucumber, lime juice, and the remaining 1 tablespoon olive oil. Season with a pinch of salt and a twist of black pepper and toss to combine.

6. Serve a black bean burger with the salad on top. See step 3 to freeze or refrigerate leftover burgers.

Day 6

Congratulations! You are halfway through The Reset. Do you feel amazing yet?

Eggs baked in avocado is one of my favorite quick breakfasts. It's a twist on the classic diner dish Toad in the Hole, but we swap the bread with avocado for a creamy, healthy upgrade. For lunch, sautéed mushrooms and flash-sautéed spinach get a big boost from a warm vinaigrette sprinkled with toasted pine nuts. Sweet roasted bell pepper becomes a wholesome, gratifying dinner when stuffed with black-eyed peas and quinoa.

Baked Eggs in Avocado
with Peppers

Day 6
Breakfast

Serves 1

1 small **avocado**

Kosher salt and freshly ground black pepper

1 tablespoon **extra-virgin olive oil**, plus more for brushing

2 large **eggs**

½ **red bell pepper**, thinly sliced

½ **jalapeño**, seeded and thinly sliced

2 tablespoons chopped **fresh cilantro**

Lime wedge

1. Slice the avocado in half, remove the pit, and scoop out enough flesh from each half to accommodate 1 egg (eat or reserve the removed avocado flesh for another use). With the palm of your hand, slightly flatten the avocado so it doesn't wobble.

2. Set a medium nonstick skillet over medium-high heat. Season the cut side of the avocado with salt and pepper, brush the flesh with the olive oil, and place it cut-side down in the skillet. Cook until it begins to brown, about 1 minute, and flip. Carefully crack an egg into each hole and season with a pinch of salt and a twist of black pepper. Reduce the heat to

medium-low, cover, and cook until the whites are set and the yolks are runny, about 4 minutes. Transfer to a plate and tent with foil.

3. Increase the heat under the skillet to medium-high, add the 1 tablespoon olive oil and heat to shimmering, then add the bell pepper and jalapeño. Season with a pinch of salt and a twist of black pepper and cook, stirring occasionally, until the vegetables soften, about 5 minutes. Remove from the heat and stir in the cilantro. Top the avocado with the peppers, garnish with a squeeze of lime, and serve.

Warm Spinach and Mushroom Salad

with Pine Nuts

Serves 1

2 tablespoons **pine nuts**

1 tablespoon **red wine vinegar**

1 teaspoon **Dijon mustard**

3 tablespoons **extra-virgin olive oil**

2 cups thinly sliced **cremini mushrooms**

3 cups **spinach leaves**

Kosher salt and freshly ground black pepper

1. Preheat the oven to 350°F.

2. Place the pine nuts on a sheet pan and cook until lightly toasted, about 8 minutes. Set aside.

3. In a small bowl, whisk together the vinegar and mustard.

4. Set a large skillet over medium-high heat. Add the olive oil and heat to shimmering, then add the mushrooms. Cook until the mushrooms begin to brown, about 5 minutes. Add the spinach, season with a pinch of salt and a twist of black pepper, and cook until the spinach begins to wilt, about 1 minute. Stir in the vinaigrette.

5. Remove from the heat, stir in the pine nuts, and serve.

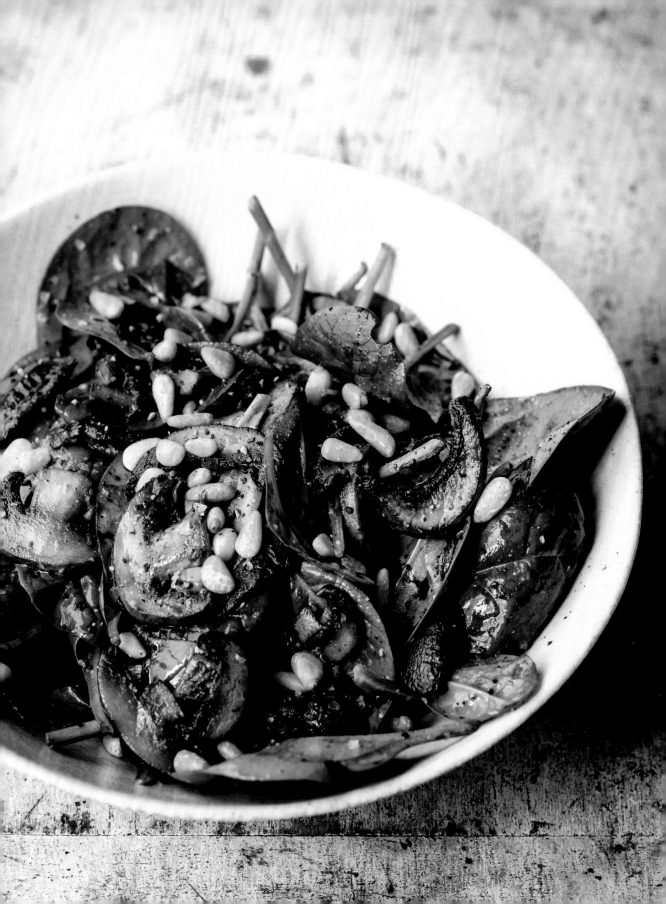

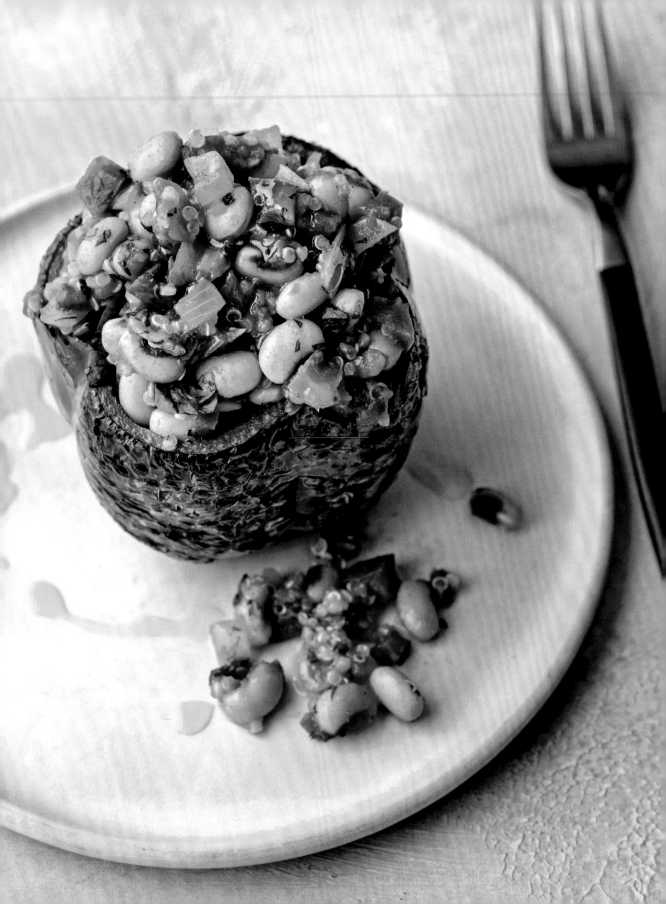

Stuffed Peppers

with Black-Eyed Peas and Quinoa

Serves 1

1 **green bell pepper**

1 tablespoon **extra-virgin olive oil**, plus more for drizzling

Kosher salt and freshly ground black pepper

1 cup **Black-Eyed Pea Stew** (from Day 5, page 43)

¼ cup **cooked Quinoa** (page 244)

Juice of ½ lime

2 tablespoons finely chopped **fresh cilantro**

1. Preheat the oven to 400°F. Line a sheet pan with foil.

2. Set the bell pepper on a cutting board and slice off the top to expose the seeds. Use a spoon to scoop out the seeds and ribs.

3. Coat the bell pepper inside and out with the olive oil, season with a pinch of salt and a twist of black pepper, and place on the lined sheet pan. Roast until the pepper begins to soften and char, about 10 minutes.

4. Meanwhile, in a medium saucepan, reheat the black-eyed pea stew over medium heat. When hot, stir in the quinoa, lime juice, and cilantro. Taste and adjust for seasoning, adding salt and pepper as needed.

5. Carefully fill the pepper with the stew, drizzle with olive oil, and serve.

Day 7

Corned beef hash is one of my all-time-favorite diner breakfasts. This lightened-up version ditches the meat, swaps the white potato for sweet, and introduces a few fistfuls of healthy kale. Lunch is a dairy-free risotto that's as indulgent as those made with butter and parmesan, while dinner is an aromatic, filling, and flavorful vegetable chili that I like to serve with extra jalapeños.

Sweet Potato and Kale Hash
with Fried Eggs

Day 7
Breakfast

Serves 1

2½ tablespoons **coconut oil**

1 medium **sweet potato**, peeled and cut into ¼-inch dice

Kosher salt and freshly ground black pepper

4 **kale leaves and tender stems**, thinly sliced (about 2 cups)

½ **red bell pepper**, cut into ¼-inch dice

1 **scallion**, finely sliced

½ teaspoon **ground cumin**

½ teaspoon **paprika**

2 large **eggs**

1. Set a large skillet over medium-high heat. Add 2 tablespoons of the coconut oil, the sweet potato, and a pinch of salt and cook until the potatoes begin to soften and brown, about 5 minutes. Add the kale, bell pepper, scallion, cumin, paprika, a pinch of salt, and a twist of black pepper and cook until the kale wilts and softens, about 5 minutes. Taste, adding salt and pepper as needed.

2. Meanwhile, in a small nonstick skillet, heat the remaining ½ tablespoon coconut oil over medium heat. When the pan is hot, carefully crack the eggs into the pan. Cover and cook until the whites are set but the yolks are still runny, about 3 minutes. Season with a pinch of salt and a twist of black pepper.

3. Top the hash with the eggs and serve.

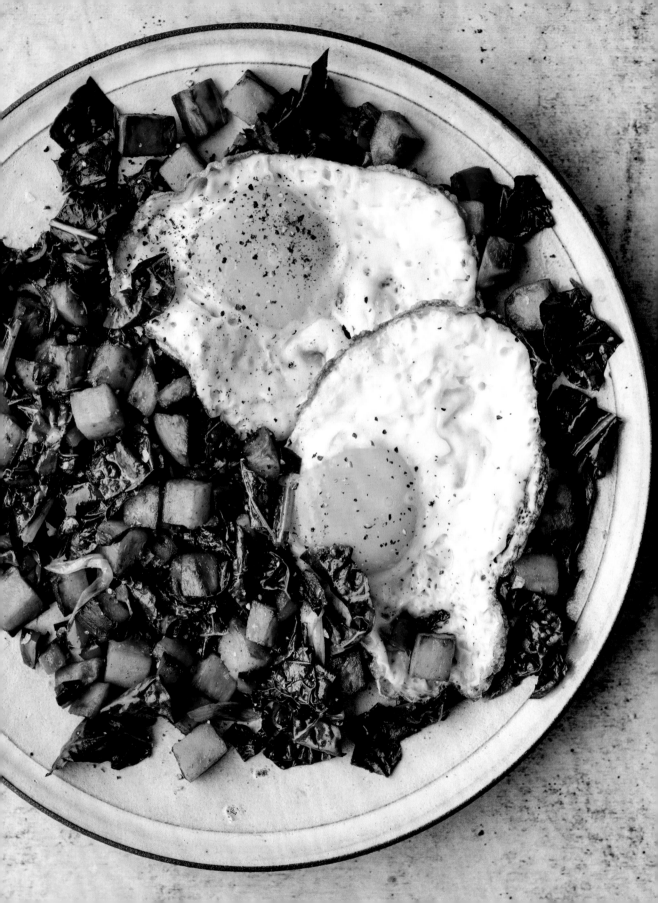

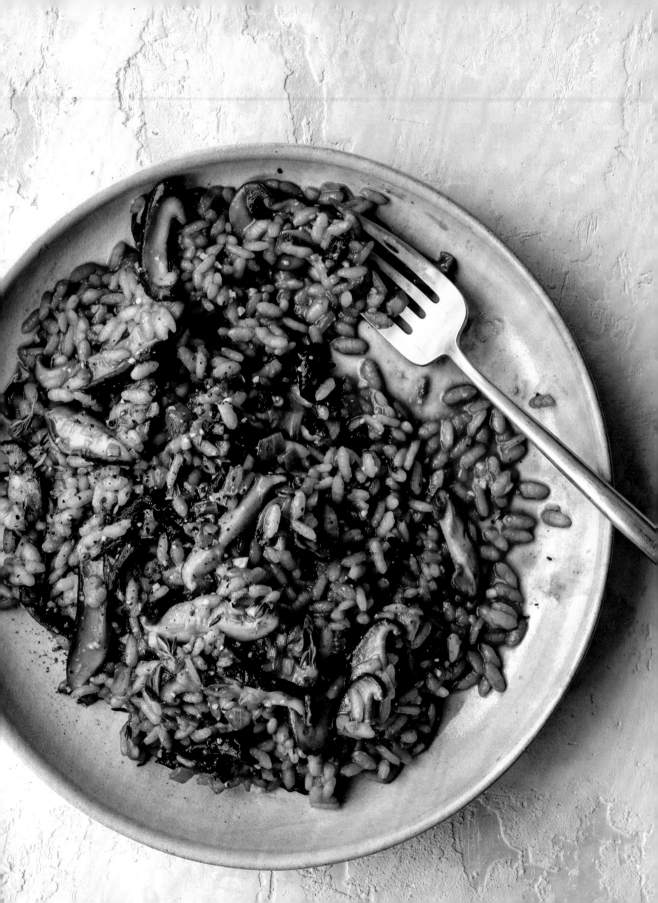

Wild Mushroom Risotto

Makes 2 servings (reserve 1 cup of risotto for the Baked Stuffed Portobellos, Day 10, page 74)

3 cups **Mushroom Stock** (page 241), or good-quality canned or boxed

3 tablespoons **extra-virgin olive oil**

1 small **yellow onion**, finely chopped

2 **garlic cloves**, minced

Kosher salt and freshly ground black pepper

3 cups thinly sliced **wild mushrooms** (such as shiitake, cremini, oyster), tough stems removed

1 teaspoon **fresh thyme leaves**, finely chopped

1 cup **Arborio rice**

¼ cup **Dairy-Free Parmesan** (page 241)

1. In a medium saucepan, warm the Mushroom Stock over medium-low heat. Adjust the heat if necessary and keep it warm until needed.

2. Place a large skillet over medium heat. Add 2 tablespoons of the olive oil and heat to shimmering, then add the onion, garlic, and a pinch of salt and twist of black pepper. Cook until the onion begins to soften, about 3 minutes. Add the remaining 1 tablespoon olive oil, the mushrooms, and thyme and cook until the mushrooms soften, release their liquid, and begin to brown, about 5 minutes.

3. Add the rice and cook, stirring occasionally, until the rice begins to toast, about 2 minutes. Add 1 ladleful of the warm stock, stirring constantly, until all of the liquid has been absorbed. Repeat this process until all but about 1 cup of the stock is incorporated and the rice is very creamy, but still slightly al dente, about 25 minutes. If you prefer softer rice, continue the process with the remaining stock.

4. Remove the saucepan from the heat, stir in the Dairy-Free Parmesan. Set aside 1 cup of risotto for the Baked Stuffed Portobellos on Day 10, page 74, then divide the rest between two plates and serve.

Vegetable Chili

Day 7
Dinner

Serves 6

¼ cup **extra-virgin olive oil**

2 medium **eggplants**, peeled and cut into ¾-inch cubes

Kosher salt and freshly ground black pepper

1 small **yellow onion**, cut into ¼-inch dice

1 **red bell pepper**, cut into ½-inch pieces

2 **garlic cloves**, minced

1 **jalapeño**, seeded and finely chopped, plus more for garnish (optional)

2 tablespoons **unsweetened cocoa powder**

5 teaspoons **chili powder**

1 tablespoon **ground cumin**

1½ teaspoons **ground coriander**

¼ teaspoon **ground cinnamon**

¼ cup **fresh oregano leaves**, finely chopped (about 1 heaping tablespoon)

1 cup **dried black-eyed peas**, soaked overnight in cold **water**

4 cups **Vegetable Stock**, homemade (page 240) or good-quality store-bought

1 (14.5- to 15-ounce) can **crushed San Marzano tomatoes**

Fresh cilantro, for serving

1. Place a large Dutch oven over medium-high heat. Add the olive oil and heat to shimmering, then add the eggplant. Cook, stirring occasionally, until the eggplant starts to brown and soften, about 8 minutes. Season with a pinch of salt and a twist of black pepper. Add the onion, bell pepper, garlic, and jalapeño and cook until the vegetables soften, about 5 minutes.

2. Stir in the cocoa powder, chili powder, cumin, coriander, cinnamon, and oregano and stir to combine. Cook, stirring constantly, for 1 minute. Add the black-eyed peas, Vegetable Stock, and crushed tomatoes and bring to a simmer. Cook, stirring occasionally, until the peas are tender, about 45 minutes.

3. Remove from the heat, taste, and add more salt and pepper if needed. Serve topped with cilantro and jalapeño, if using.

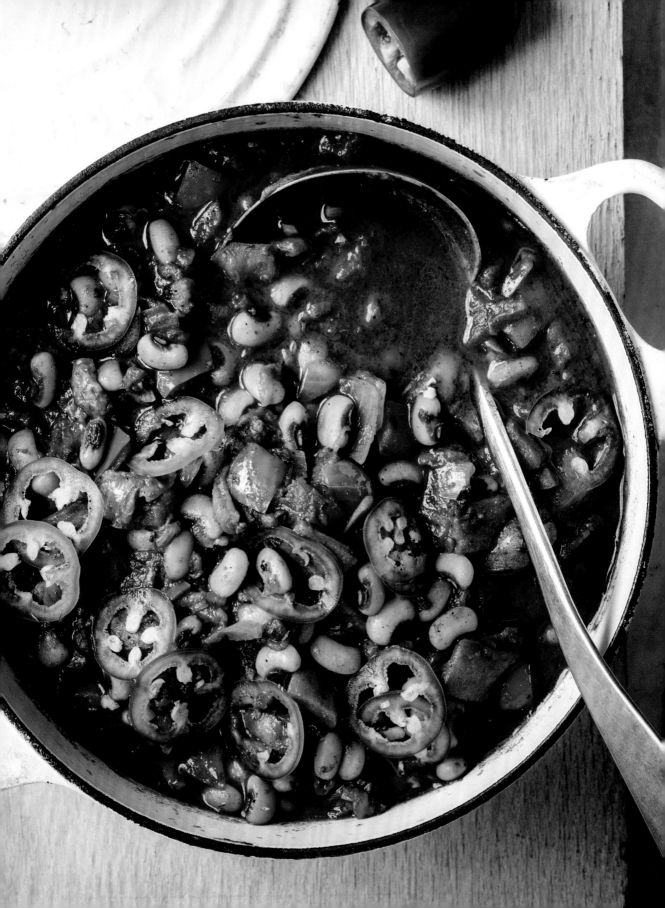

Day 8

The key to wonderful scrambled eggs is to cook them gently and briefly, coddling them until they are just set. Here, we fold the warm, custardy eggs with bright, cool vegetables and herbs for a brilliant yin and yang. Something magical happens when you combine chickpeas, sweet potato, and coconut milk and stew them as we do for today's lunch. As with grilled portobello mushrooms, grilled cauliflower steaks make a remarkable substitute for meat, especially when spice-coated and charred.

Avocado and Tomato Egg Scramble

Day 8
Breakfast

Serves 1

1 tablespoon **extra-virgin olive oil**

3 large **eggs**, beaten

Kosher salt and freshly ground black pepper

½ **avocado**, diced

¼ cup halved **grape tomatoes**

2 tablespoons finely chopped **fresh cilantro**

1. Set a large nonstick skillet over medium heat. Add the olive oil and heat to shimmering. Add the eggs and cook, occasionally stirring with a silicone spatula, until the eggs just begin to set, about 2 minutes.

2. Season with a pinch of salt and a twist of black pepper and remove the pan from the heat. Stir in the avocado, tomatoes, and cilantro and serve.

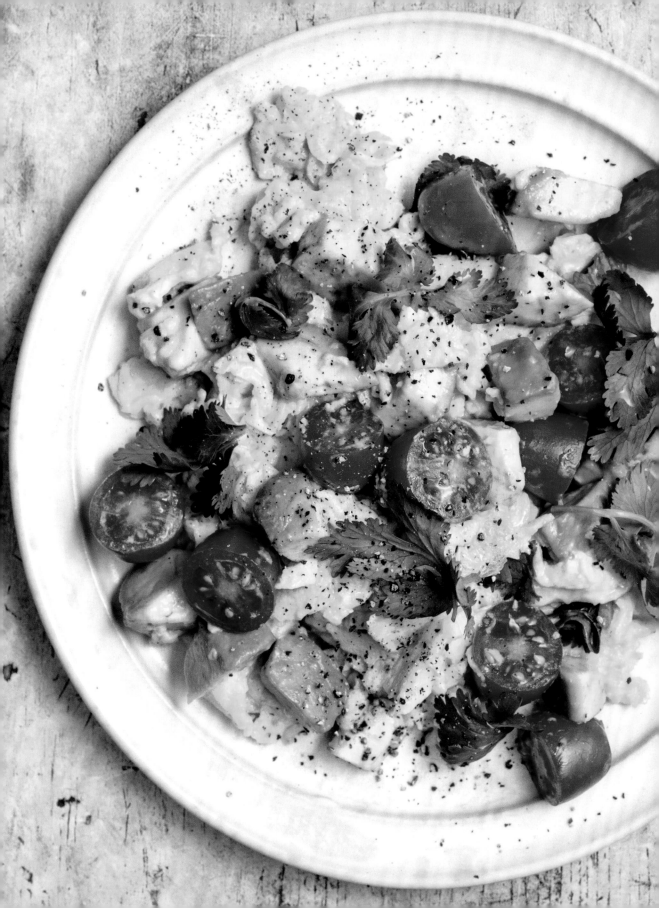

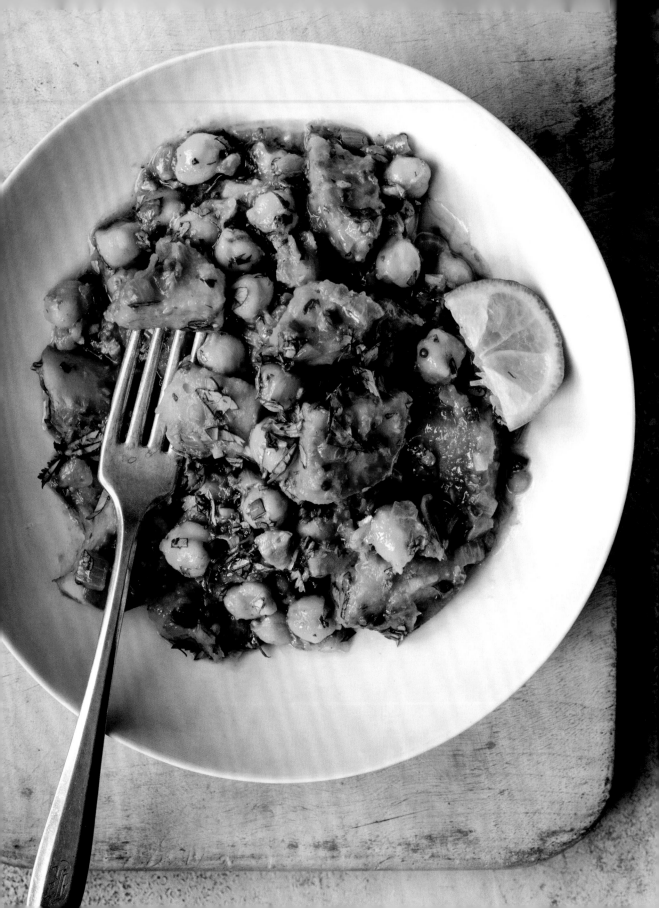

Sweet Potato and Coconut Stew

Serves 1

2 tablespoons **coconut oil**

1 medium **sweet potato**, peeled and cut into 1-inch cubes

Kosher salt and freshly ground black pepper

1 small **yellow onion**, cut into ¼-inch dice

1 **garlic clove**, minced

1 **jalapeño**, seeded and finely chopped

2-inch piece **fresh ginger**, peeled and grated

1 teaspoon **ground coriander**

½ cup **Vegetable Stock**, homemade (page 240) or good-quality store-bought

½ cup **unsweetened full-fat coconut milk**

½ cup **cooked chickpeas**, drained and rinsed if using canned

1 tablespoon finely chopped **fresh cilantro**

Lime wedge

1. Set a medium saucepan over medium-high heat. Add the coconut oil, sweet potato, and a pinch of salt and a twist of black pepper and cook until the potatoes begin to soften and brown, about 5 minutes. Reduce the heat to medium-low.

2. Add the onion, garlic, jalapeño, ginger, and coriander and cook until the onion softens and the mixture is very fragrant, about 3 minutes.

3. Add the Vegetable Stock, coconut milk, and chickpeas and bring to a simmer. Cook, stirring occasionally, until the sweet potatoes are very tender and the liquid has reduced and thickened, about 20 minutes.

4. Remove from the heat, stir in the cilantro, and spoon into a bowl. Serve with a squeeze of lime.

Grilled Spiced Cauliflower Steaks

with Jeweled Rice

Serves 1

1 head of **cauliflower**

3 tablespoons **extra-virgin olive oil**, plus more for drizzling

2 **garlic cloves**, minced

1 tablespoon grated **fresh ginger**

1 teaspoon **curry powder**

Grated zest and juice of 1 lime

Kosher salt

1 cup cooked **Brown Rice** (page 248)

2 tablespoons **golden raisins**

1 tablespoon finely chopped **fresh cilantro**

1. To prepare the cauliflower steak, remove the leaves and all but 1 inch of stem from the head. Place the head stem-side down on the cutting board. With a heavy, sharp knife, slice a 1-inch "steak" from the middle of the head. Reserve the rest of the cauliflower for another use.

2. Preheat a grill or grill pan to medium-high heat.

3. In a medium bowl, whisk together the olive oil, garlic, ginger, curry powder, lime zest, and lime juice. Season with salt.

4. Use a silicone brush to coat both sides of the cauliflower steak with the spice paste. Place the cauliflower on the grill and cook until it chars and begins to soften, about 8 minutes. Use a spatula to flip the cauliflower over and grill until the second side is charred, about 8 minutes more.

5. Meanwhile, in a medium bowl, stir together the rice, raisins, and cilantro. Mound the rice on a plate, top with the cauliflower, drizzle with olive oil, and serve.

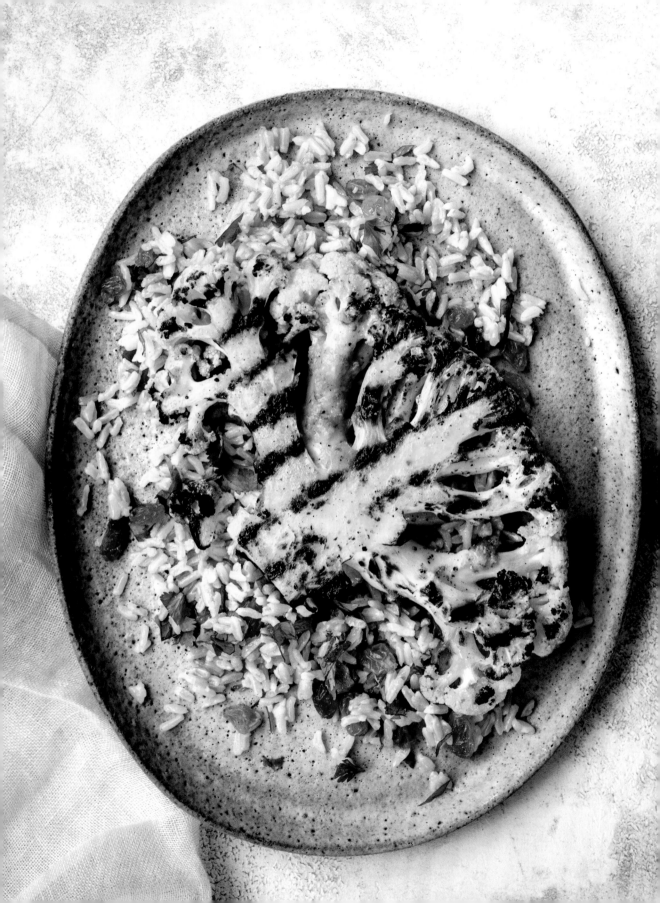

Day 9

I know toasting nuts is an extra step, but it makes all the difference in simple breakfasts like this one. The nuts get nuttier, crispier, and more aromatic. Lunch features thin slices of crunchy apple set against silky-soft roasted squash, all tossed into an elegant salad. Serve anything over brown rice, such as mixed veggies in a ginger-garlic-soy sauce like we do for dinner, and it instantly becomes comfort food.

Oatmeal
with Coconut Cream, Strawberries, and Toasted Almonds

Day 9
Breakfast

Serves 1

¼ cup **slivered almonds**

1 tablespoon **coconut oil**

⅓ cup **steel-cut oats**

½ cup **coconut cream** (not cream of coconut)

Kosher salt

6 **strawberries**, hulled and sliced

1. Preheat the oven to 350°F.

2. Spread the almonds on a sheet pan and cook until lightly toasted, about 8 minutes. Set aside.

3. Set a medium saucepan over medium heat. Add the coconut oil and the oats and cook, stirring occasionally, until the oats are fragrant, about 1 minute. Add the coconut cream, ¾ cup water, and a pinch of salt. Bring to a simmer and cook, partially covered and stirring occasionally, until the oats are tender, about 45 minutes.

4. Remove the oats from the heat, stir in the strawberries, top with toasted almonds, and serve.

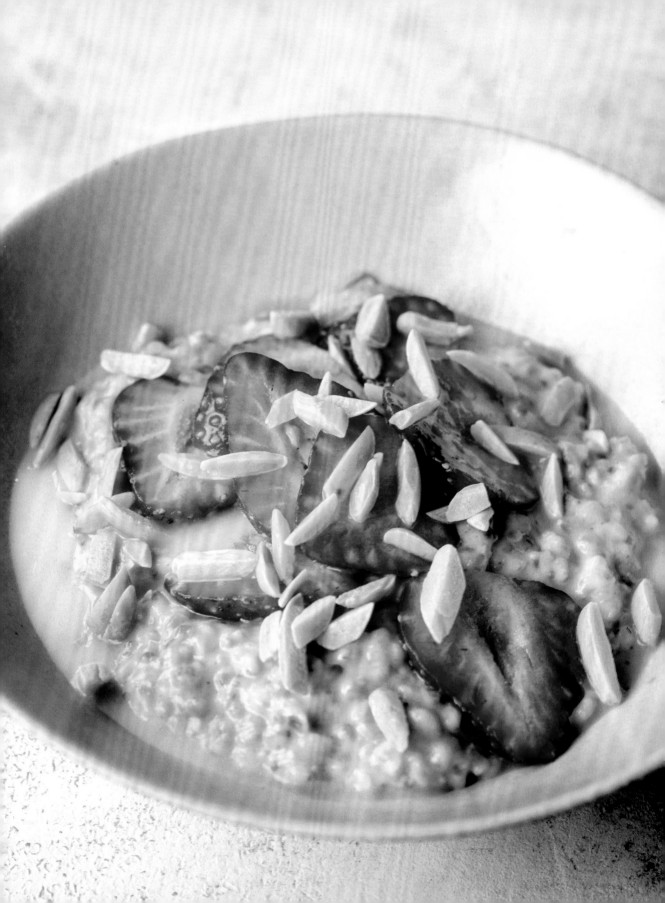

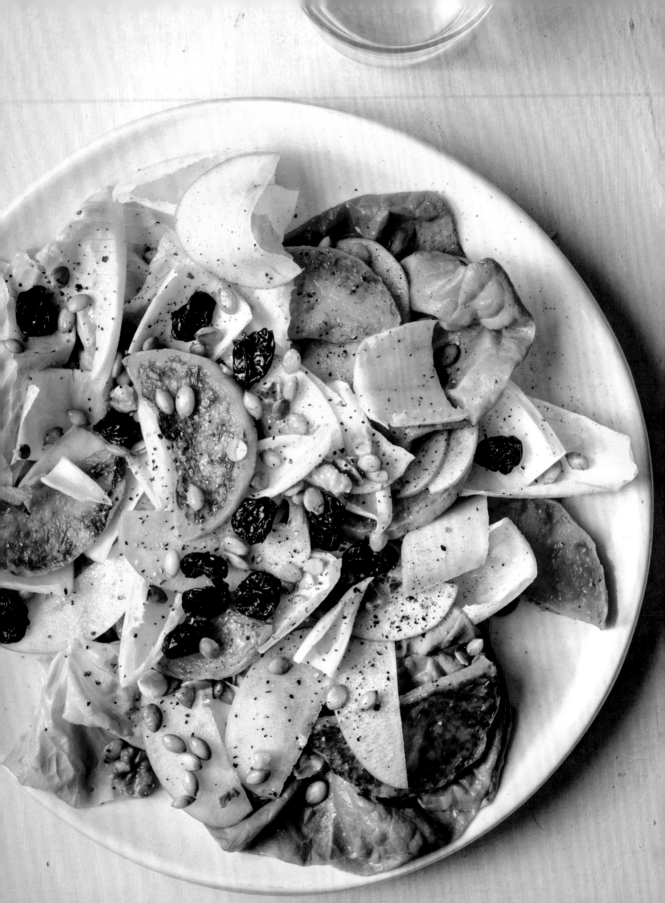

Bibb Salad

with Apples, Squash, and Walnuts

Serves 2

¼ cup **walnut halves**

½ small **butternut squash**, seeded and cut into ½-inch-thick slices (use the other half for the Stuffed Butternut Squash, page 40)

4 tablespoons **extra-virgin olive oil**

Kosher salt and freshly ground black pepper

3 tablespoons **apple cider vinegar**

1 small head **Bibb lettuce**, cored and torn into 1-inch pieces

1 small head **Belgian endive**, cored and cut crosswise into 1-inch pieces

½ **Granny Smith apple**, unpeeled, cored, and thinly sliced

2 tablespoons **dried cherries**

1 tablespoon **roasted pumpkin seeds** (pepitas)

1. Preheat the oven to 350°F.

2. Arrange the walnuts on a sheet pan and cook until lightly toasted, about 8 minutes. Transfer the walnuts to a cutting board and when cool enough to handle, roughly chop and set aside.

3. Increase the oven temperature to 425°F. Line a sheet pan with foil.

4. Arrange the squash on the lined sheet pan. Coat the exposed flesh with 1 tablespoon of the olive oil, season with a pinch of salt and a twist of black pepper, and cook until tender, about 20 minutes.

5. Meanwhile, in a large bowl, whisk together the remaining 3 tablespoons olive oil and the vinegar. Season with a pinch of salt and a twist of black pepper.

6. Add the lettuce, endive, apple, toasted walnuts, and roasted squash slices to the dressing and toss to coat. Divide the salad between two plates. Garnish with cherries and roasted pumpkin seeds and serve.

Veggie Stir-Fry over Brown Rice

Serves 1

3 tablespoons **tamari** (wheat-free soy sauce)

1 tablespoon finely grated **fresh ginger**

1 **garlic clove**, minced

3 tablespoons **extra-virgin olive oil**

1 stalk **asparagus**, tough end removed, stalk sliced into 2-inch pieces

1 medium **carrot**, thinly sliced

½ **bell pepper** (any color), thinly sliced

½ cup **cauliflower** florets

½ medium **zucchini**, thinly sliced

Kosher salt and freshly ground black pepper

½ cup cooked **Brown Rice** (page 248), warmed

1. In a medium bowl, whisk together the tamari, ginger, and garlic. Set aside.

2. Set a large skillet over medium-high heat. Add the olive oil and heat to shimmering, then add the asparagus, carrot, bell pepper, cauliflower, and zucchini. Season lightly with salt and pepper and cook, stirring occasionally, until the vegetables are soft and slightly browned, about 10 minutes.

3. Transfer the vegetables to the bowl with the tamari mixture and toss to combine. Serve over the brown rice.

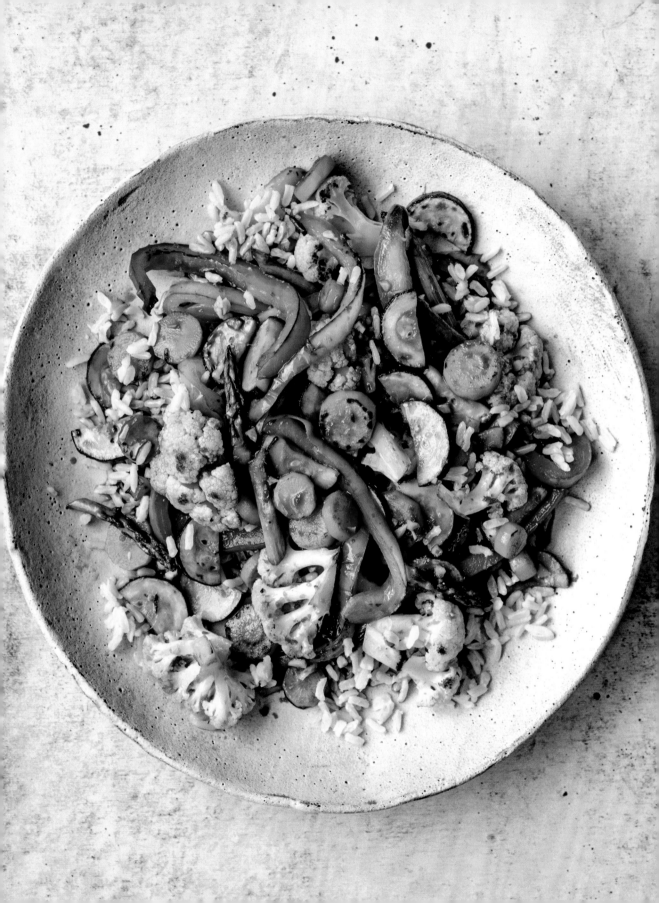

Day 10

Congrats, friends, today is the last day of The Reset! We kick off the morning with an easy, breezy, tropical smoothie and roll into lunch with a brilliant shaved Brussels sprouts, apple, and brown rice salad. For dinner, the last meal of the 10-Day Reset, we go back to those meaty, savory, satisfying portobellos, but this time we load them up with our leftover Wild Mushroom Risotto (page 55) from Day 7. Cheers!

Almond, Berry, and Chia Smoothie
with Spinach

Day 10
Breakfast

Serves 1

1 cup fresh or frozen **strawberries**

1 cup **unsweetened almond milk**

1 tablespoon **chia seeds**

2 cups **spinach leaves**

1 small peeled **banana** (fresh or frozen)

1 **orange**, peeled and chopped

Juice of 1 lemon

In a blender, combine all of the ingredients and process until smooth.

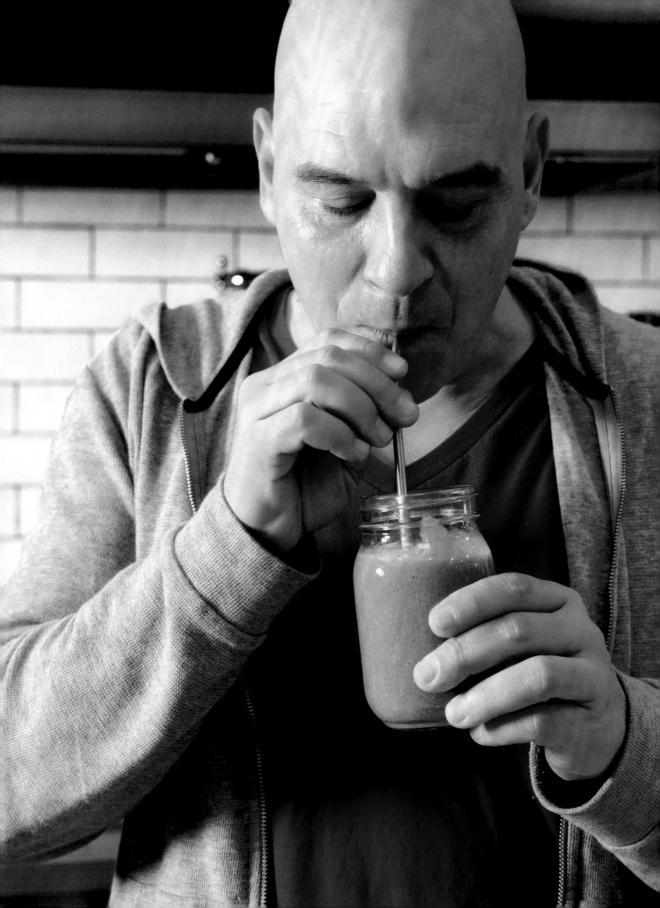

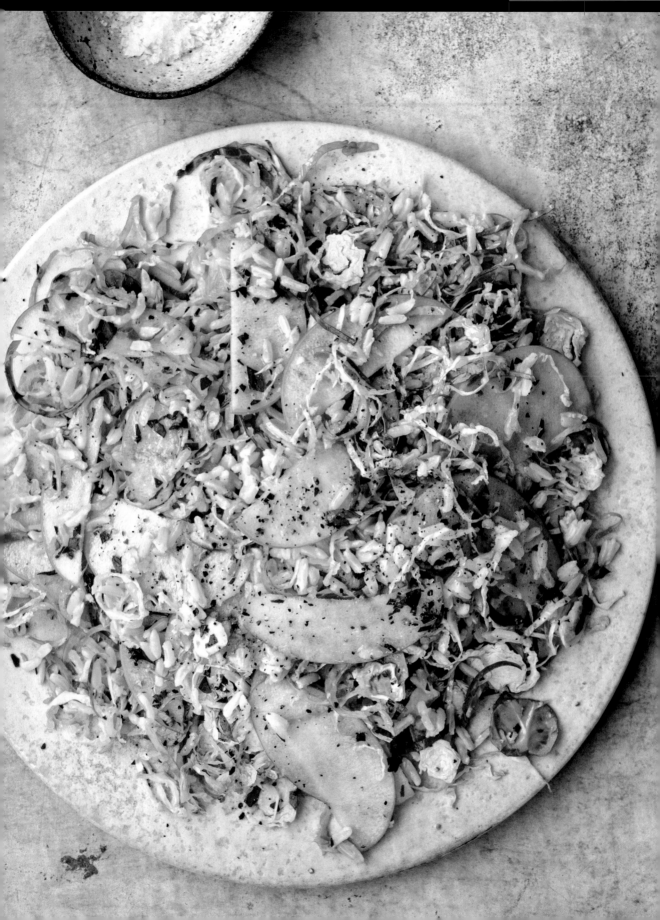

Brussels Sprouts, Apple, and Brown Rice Salad

Day 10
Lunch

Serves 1

3 tablespoons **extra-virgin olive oil**

3 tablespoons **apple cider vinegar**

Juice of ½ lemon

1 teaspoon **Dijon mustard**

1 tablespoon grated **fresh ginger**

Kosher salt and freshly ground black pepper

2 cups **Brussels sprouts**

½ **Granny Smith apple**, unpeeled, cored, and thinly sliced

½ cup cooked **Brown Rice** (page 248), at room temperature

1 tablespoon finely chopped **fresh flat-leaf parsley**

1. In a medium bowl, whisk together the olive oil, vinegar, lemon juice, mustard, and ginger. Season with a pinch of salt and a twist of black pepper.

2. To shave the Brussels sprouts, use a food processor fitted with the slicing blade, a mandoline, or a very sharp knife and a steady hand. Add the shaved Brussels sprouts to the bowl with the vinaigrette.

3. To the shaved Brussels sprouts, add the apple, brown rice, and parsley and toss together. Taste and add salt and pepper if needed.

Baked Stuffed Portobellos

Day 10
Dinner

Serves 1

2 tablespoons **pine nuts**

2 **portobello mushroom caps**, stems and gills removed

2 tablespoons **extra-virgin olive oil**, plus more for serving

Kosher salt and freshly ground black pepper

1 cup **Wild Mushroom Risotto** (from Day 7, page 55)

1 large **egg**, beaten

2 tablespoons finely chopped **fresh flat-leaf parsley**

2 tablespoons **Dairy-Free Parmesan** (page 241), plus more for serving

1. Preheat the oven to 350°F.

2. Set the pine nuts on a sheet pan and cook until lightly toasted, about 8 minutes. Set aside.

3. Increase the oven temperature to 425°F. Place the mushrooms gill-side down on a sheet pan, drizzle with the olive oil, and season with a pinch of salt and a twist of black pepper. Roast them until browned and softened, about 12 minutes.

4. Meanwhile, in a medium bowl, combine the wild mushroom risotto, egg, parsley, and toasted pine nuts and stir to combine.

5. Remove the mushrooms from the oven, flip, and top each cap with ½ cup of the risotto mixture. Top with the Dairy-Free Parmesan, return to the oven, and cook until the risotto is warmed through, about 15 minutes.

6. Drizzle with olive oil, sprinkle with more dairy-free parmesan, and serve.

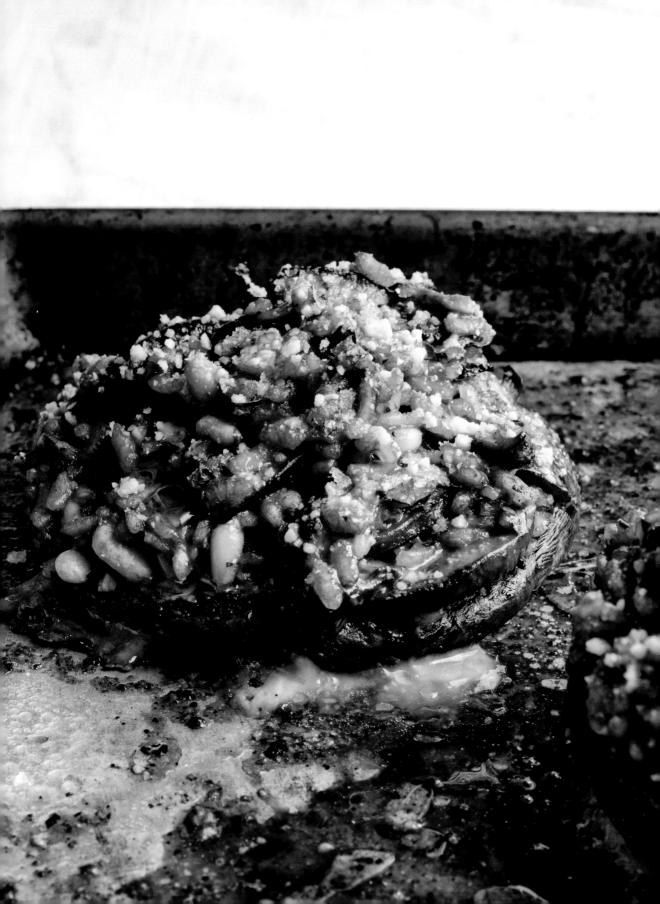

Dairy-Free Fix

I don't want to live in a world without dairy—it's my favorite food group! To me, there is nothing better than creamy Greek yogurt, stinky cheeses, and butterfat-filled ice cream. Unfortunately, dairy is one of my worst triggers and I really pay for it the day after indulging. Imagine a horrible college hangover combined with being woken up to someone hitting your hands, knees, and elbows with a hammer. That about sums it up!

So I worked really hard to come up with recipes that will help me avoid using cow's milk, butter, and cheese without feeling like I'm missing out. Some recipes rely on ingredients like oat milk, cashew milk, coconut milk, and nutritional yeast to provide the texture, flavor, and satisfaction of dairy foods without the guilt or pain. (Seriously, the Dairy-Free Parmesan recipe in the pantry chapter on page 241 will change your life.) Other recipes in this chapter just skip the dairy (and nondairy alternatives) altogether—the recipes are so delicious that you won't even miss it.

As hard as I try to be perfect, let's face it—I'm only human, which means that there will be days when I make a big bowl of ice cream disappear faster than a snowman in Phoenix. But I make the decision with the understanding that I'll pay for it on the other side. That's why I said in the beginning that this book is a guide, not a bible. There are going to be times when you slip, stumble, and cheat, but at least you'll do so knowingly and armed with recipes to get you back on track to feeling great.

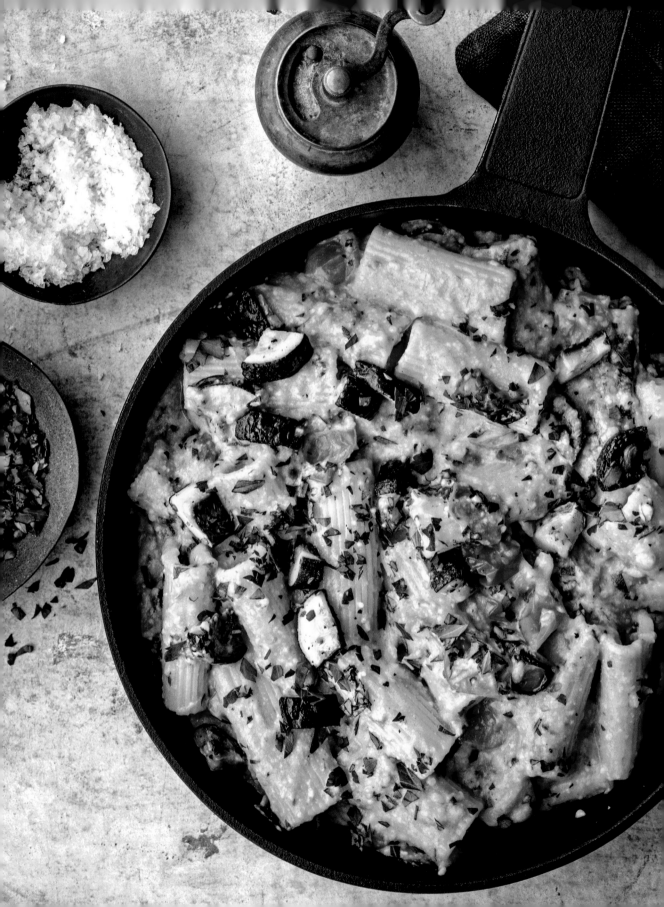

Roasted Vegetable Mac and Cheese

Serves 4

Kosher salt and freshly ground
   black pepper

½ pound **rigatoni**

1 **zucchini**, quartered lengthwise and
   sliced crosswise to ½-inch-thick
   pieces

1 pint **cherry tomatoes**, halved

6 tablespoons **extra-virgin olive oil**

2 **garlic cloves**, minced

¼ cup **unbleached, nonbromated
   flour**

2½ cups **unsweetened cashew or
   oat milk**

Dairy-Free Parmesan (page 241)

1 tablespoon **hot sauce**, plus more
   to taste

¼ cup chopped **fresh flat-leaf
   parsley**, plus more for garnish

People are more obsessed with my mac and cheese recipes than almost any other dish. That's because I load mine up with various cheeses and heavy cream to create the ultimate comfort food. But what do you do if you're trying to avoid dairy like me? You labor to come up with a recipe that will scratch that comfort-food itch while steering clear of cheese. And that's what I've done here by using my Dairy-Free Parmesan (page 241). Prepare to be blown away!

1. Preheat the oven to 500°F.

2. Add 3 tablespoons of salt to a large pot of water and bring to a boil over high heat. Add the pasta and cook until just al dente, about 1 minute less than the package directions. Drain and set aside.

3. In a large bowl, toss together the zucchini, tomatoes, and 2 tablespoons of the olive oil. Season with a pinch of salt and a twist of black pepper. Arrange in a single layer on a sheet pan and roast in the hot oven until the vegetables are nicely charred, about 10 minutes. Set the sheet pan aside.

4. Place a large heavy-bottomed skillet over medium heat. Add the remaining 4 tablespoons olive oil and heat to shimmering, then add the garlic. Cook until aromatic, about 2 minutes. Add the flour and whisk to combine until a sandy mixture forms, about 1 minute. Slowly add the cashew milk while whisking until the mixture is smooth. Cook until the sauce comes to a simmer and thickens, whisking the entire time, about 5 minutes.

5. Add the Dairy-Free Parmesan and hot sauce to the skillet and whisk to combine. Season with a pinch of salt and a twist of black pepper. Add the roasted vegetables, drained rigatoni, and parsley and stir to combine. Taste and adjust for seasoning, adding salt, pepper, and hot sauce as needed. Garnish with parsley and serve.

Cream of Wild Mushroom and Barley Soup

Serves 6

¼ cup **extra-virgin olive oil**

1 medium **red onion**, finely chopped

2 **garlic cloves**, minced

Kosher salt and freshly ground black pepper

5 cups thinly sliced **cremini mushrooms**

2 tablespoons finely chopped **fresh rosemary**

¼ cup **unbleached, nonbromated flour**

½ cup **dry red wine**

4 cups **Beef Bone Broth** (page 237)

1 cup **pearled barley**

1 cup **unsweetened oat milk**

Fresh dill, for garnish

Bone broth is like beef stock on steroids, and it elevates any recipe that it's added to. Not only does it provide a deep, rich flavor boost, it also brings great health benefits from all those vitamins, minerals, and collagen that fight inflammation, aid digestion, and maybe even help to prevent colds! Oat milk adds the silky texture of real dairy—if you haven't cooked with it before, be prepared to be pleasantly surprised—it's slightly sweet and pleasantly earthy. Take my word for it, this soup is every bit as creamy and comforting as one made with cream.

1. Place a large heavy-bottomed skillet over medium heat. Add the olive oil and heat to shimmering, then add the onion, garlic, and a pinch of salt. Cook until aromatic and just starting to soften, about 2 minutes.

2. Add the mushrooms and rosemary and cook, stirring occasionally, until the mushrooms have given up most of their liquid and are beginning to brown, about 5 minutes.

3. Add the flour and cook for 1 minute, stirring constantly. Add the red wine and bone broth to deglaze the pan, scraping with a wooden spoon to loosen the browned bits on the bottom. Bring to a boil and then reduce the heat to medium-low to maintain a gentle simmer. Add the barley and cook, stirring occasionally, until it's almost tender, about 45 minutes.

4. Taste and add salt and pepper if needed. Stir in the oat milk and continue cooking until the barley is completely tender, about 15 minutes longer. Garnish with dill and serve.

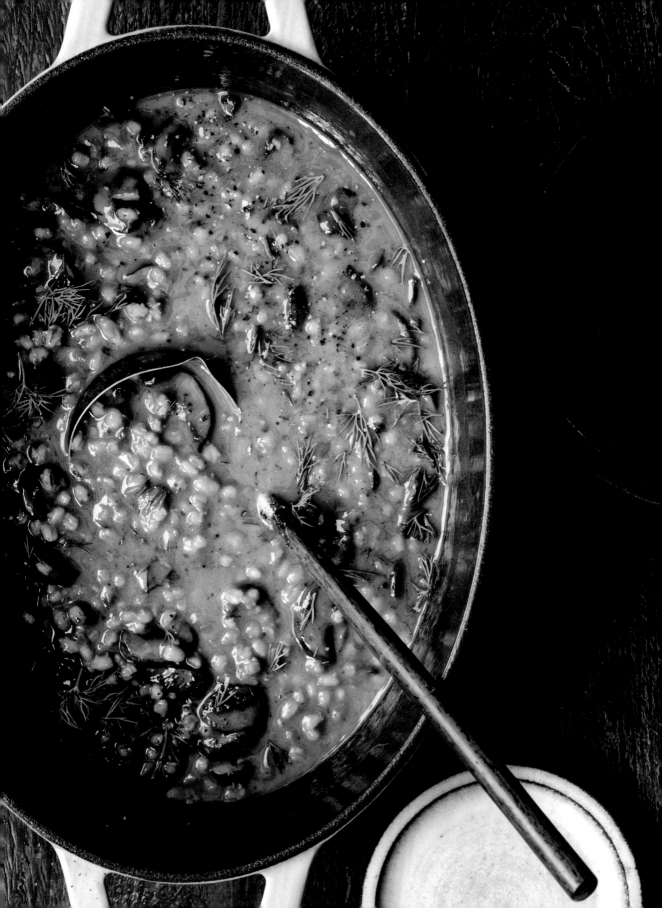

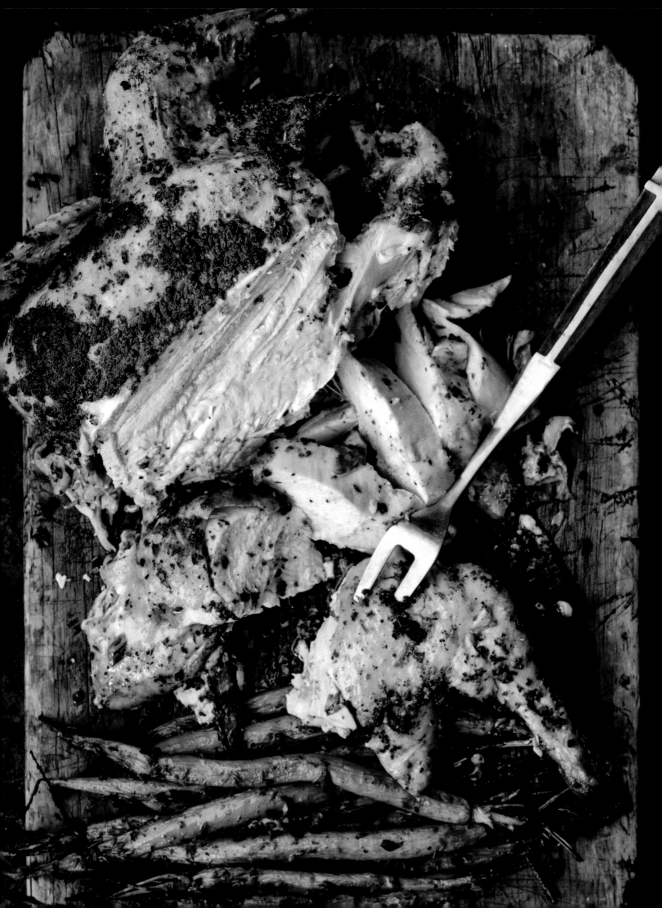

Ginger and Chile Roasted Chicken

Serves 4

1 large **chicken** (4 to 6 pounds), preferably organic

Kosher salt and freshly ground black pepper

½ cup roughly chopped peeled **fresh ginger**

1 **jalapeño**, thinly sliced into rings

¼ cup **extra-virgin olive oil**

½ cup **fresh cilantro leaves** and thin tender stems

Juice of 1 lime

I don't think I've written a cookbook without including at least one recipe for whole roasted chicken. That's because I don't think I've made it through a single week without making one at home. Properly done, there's nothing better. One of the easiest ways to achieve roast chicken greatness is to season the bird inside and out and let it marinate with the rub for as long as you can, ideally overnight (but 2 or 3 hours will do). I know most recipes say to cook chicken for a while at 350°F, but I prefer a hotter oven for a shorter amount of time because it makes incredibly crispy skin without needing to rub the skin with butter. This recipe goes great with Roasted Carrots with Cumin and Cinnamon (page 97) and Kyle's Coconut Rice (page 106).

1. Pat the chicken dry with paper towels, liberally season inside and out with salt, and refrigerate uncovered for at least 2 hours or preferably overnight.

2. Remove the chicken from the refrigerator and allow it to come to room temperature, about 30 minutes while you preheat the oven to 450°F.

3. In a blender or food processor, combine the ginger, jalapeño, olive oil, cilantro, and lime juice and process until smooth. Coat the inside and outside of the chicken with the ginger paste, and then season the inside and outside with a pinch more salt and a few twists of black pepper.

4. Roast the chicken on a sheet pan until the thickest portion of the thigh reaches an internal temperature of 160°F, about 1 hour. Midway through the cooking, and again when it's done, use a spoon to baste the chicken with any pan juices.

5. Transfer the chicken to a cutting board and let rest for 10 minutes before carving and serving.

Grilled Mahi Mahi

Serves 4

3 tablespoons **extra-virgin olive oil**

2 tablespoons finely chopped **fresh mint**

2 tablespoons **Curry Paste** (page 248) or store-bought curry powder

Juice of 1 orange

4 **skinless mahi mahi fillets** (8 ounces each)

Kosher salt and freshly ground black pepper

This is a great weekday dinner that takes minimal prep and planning to pull off. If you feel adventurous, go ahead and make your own curry paste—you'll be amazed with the results. By buying fresh, whole spices and toasting and grinding them yourself, you unleash a bounty of flavors and aromas just not present in store-bought concoctions. That said, there's no shame in buying high-quality curry powder to use in place of homemade paste—just make sure it includes ground turmeric (most curry blends do), which is great at fighting inflammation. Pair this with Roasted Pineapple and Pepper Salad (page 111) for a tropical feast.

1. In a small bowl, whisk together 2 tablespoons of the olive oil, the mint, curry paste, and half of the orange juice. Use paper towels to pat the fish fillets dry. Place the fish in a gallon-size zip-top bag, add the marinade, and refrigerate for up to 1 hour.

2. Preheat a grill or grill pan to high heat.

3. Remove the fish from the bag and place on a wire rack positioned on a sheet pan for a few minutes to allow most of the marinade to drip off. Discard the excess marinade in the bag. Drizzle the fish with the remaining 1 tablespoon olive oil and season with a few pinches of salt and twists of black pepper.

4. Transfer the fish to the grill, cover, and cook until the fish begins to char, about 5 minutes. Use a spatula to carefully flip the fish, cover, and continue grilling until cooked through, about 3 minutes. Remove the fish to a platter and drizzle with the remaining orange juice and serve.

Grilled Chicken Paillard

Serves 4

4 **boneless, skin-on chicken breast halves** (6 ounces each)

¼ cup **extra-virgin olive oil**

Grated zest and juice of 1 lemon

2 tablespoons finely chopped **fresh oregano**

Kosher salt and freshly ground black pepper

The hardest part of this recipe is flattening the chicken, and that's not hard at all! By pounding out the meat you decrease cooking time, increase surface area for more flavorful charring, and guarantee even cooking throughout the breast. (If your butcher or grocery sells pre-pounded cutlets, by all means go for it!) Sometimes simple is best, and this straightforward marinade provides a nice lemony boost to the meat. I leave the skin on because I love the flavor it brings to the table, but if you are counting calories, or just don't like it, you can certainly make this dish with skinless breasts. These go great with almost any salad, but especially the Brussels Sprouts, Apple, and Brown Rice Salad (page 73).

1. Place a chicken breast skin-side up on a large sheet of plastic wrap and cover with a second sheet. Use a meat mallet to pound the chicken to an even ¼-inch thickness. Place the breast in a gallon-size zip-top bag and repeat with the other breasts.

2. In a medium bowl, whisk together the olive oil, lemon zest, lemon juice, and oregano. Pour the marinade over the chicken and refrigerate for up to 1 hour.

3. Preheat a grill or grill pan to medium-high heat.

4. Remove the chicken from the marinade, season both sides with salt and pepper, place on the grill skin-side down, and cook, covered, until nicely charred, about 3 minutes. Flip the chicken and continue cooking, covered, until the other side is also nicely charred, about 3 minutes. Serve immediately.

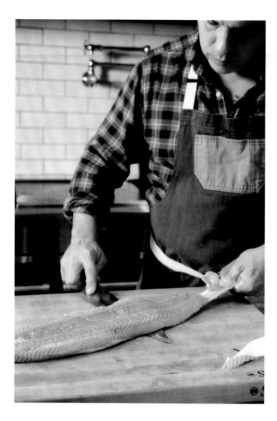
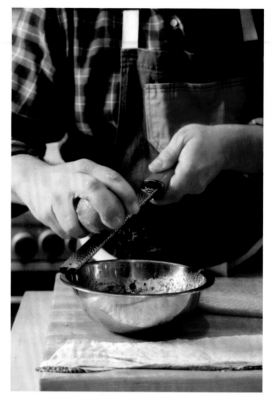
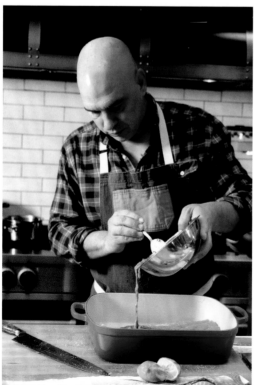
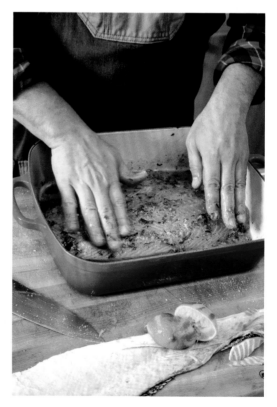

Slow-Roasted Salmon

Serves 6

3 tablespoons **extra-virgin olive oil**

3 tablespoons **raw honey**

2 tablespoons **rice vinegar**

2 tablespoons **Dijon mustard**

Grated zest and juice of 1 lime

1 tablespoon grated **fresh ginger**

¼ cup finely chopped **fresh flat-leaf parsley**

1 tablespoon **freshly ground black pepper**

Big pinch of **kosher salt**

1 side **wild salmon**, pin bones removed (about 2½ pounds)

This isn't your typical salmon—or fish—recipe. The goal isn't crispy skin accomplished in a screaming-hot skillet, or gently charred and smoky flesh cooked over charcoal, but rather succulent, buttery salmon enveloped in a slightly sweet and tangy glaze. By giving the marinade time to stick and dry, and cooking the salmon low and slow in a moderate oven, you end up with the sexiest salmon ever—proof that you don't need dairy to achieve a buttery texture. Make a batch of Kyle's Coconut Rice (page 106) or Spring Pea Hummus (page 220) to go with it.

1. In a medium bowl, whisk together the olive oil, honey, vinegar, mustard, lime zest, lime juice, ginger, parsley, black pepper, and salt.

2. Place the salmon in a 9 × 13-inch baking dish, evenly coat both sides with the marinade, and refrigerate uncovered for 1 to 2 hours.

3. Preheat the oven to 300°F.

4. Cook the fish until the thickest part reaches an internal temperature of 110°F for medium-rare, about 30 minutes. If you prefer your fish done medium, continue cooking for another 10 minutes.

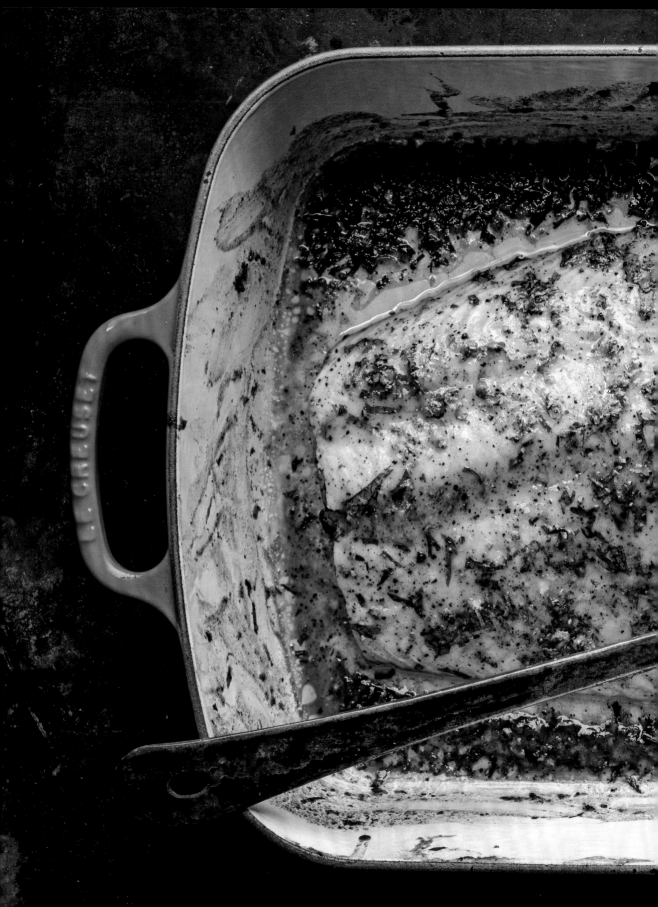

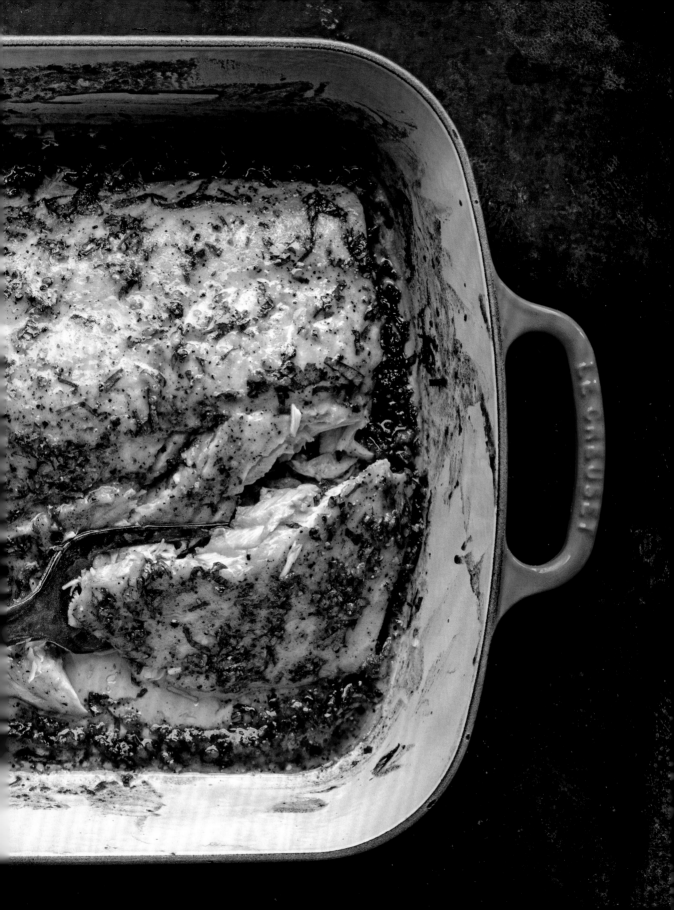

Grilled Skirt Steak with Cherry-Balsamic Sauce

Serves 6

¼ cup **extra-virgin olive oil**

¼ cup **tart cherry juice**

2 tablespoons **balsamic vinegar**

1 tablespoon chopped **fresh rosemary**

2 **garlic cloves**, minced

2 pounds **skirt steak**, trimmed of silver skin

Kosher salt and freshly ground black pepper

After rib eye, skirt steak is my favorite piece of meat for grilling. It has such an intensely beefy flavor and satisfying texture. Just make sure that you don't cook it much past medium-rare and that you slice it against the grain to keep it from getting overly chewy. In place of the customary butter-enriched pan sauce, I use the leftover marinade to create a quick, light sauce that gets sweetness and zip from cherry juice and balsamic vinegar. For a perfect bistro meal, serve this with Warm Spinach and Mushroom Salad with Pine Nuts (page 48).

1. In a small bowl, mix together the olive oil, cherry juice, vinegar, rosemary, and garlic.

2. Using paper towels, pat the steak dry. Place the meat in a gallon-size zip-top bag, add the cherry juice marinade, and refrigerate for 2 to 4 hours, occasionally moving the meat around in the bag.

3. Preheat a grill or grill pan to medium-high heat.

4. Remove the steak from the bag and place it on a wire rack positioned on a sheet pan for a few minutes to allow most of the marinade to drip off. Pour any remaining marinade from the bag and the sheet pan into a small saucepan and set aside.

5. Liberally season both sides of the steak with salt and pepper, place on the grill, and cook, uncovered, until nicely charred, about 3 minutes. Flip the steak and continue cooking uncovered until the meat is medium-rare and the other side is also nicely charred, about 3 minutes.

6. While the second side is cooking, place the saucepan containing the leftover marinade over high heat, bring to a boil, and then remove from the heat.

7. When the steak is done, remove it to a platter and let rest for 5 minutes before thinly slicing the meat against the grain. Serve with the cherry sauce.

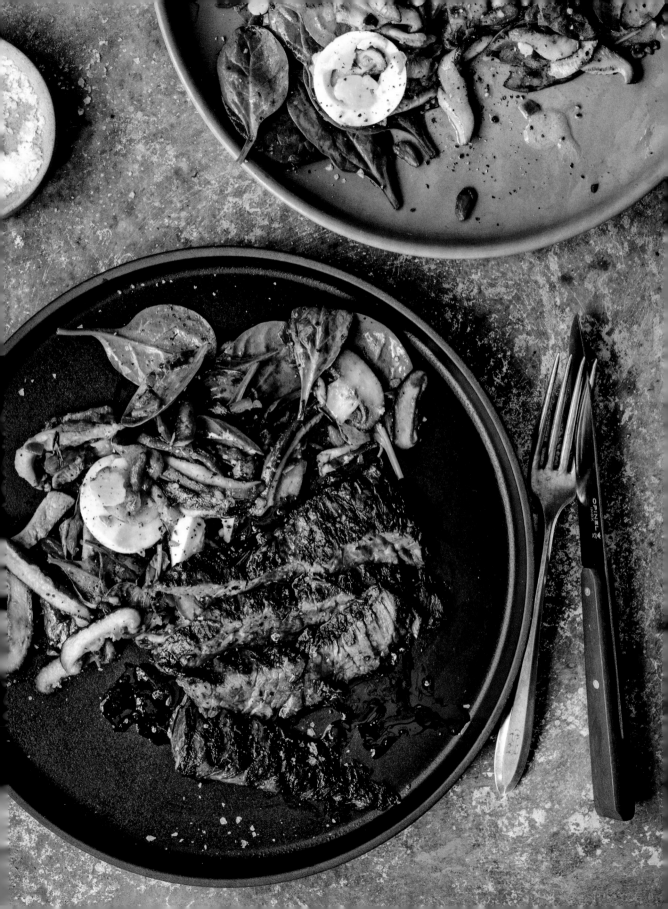

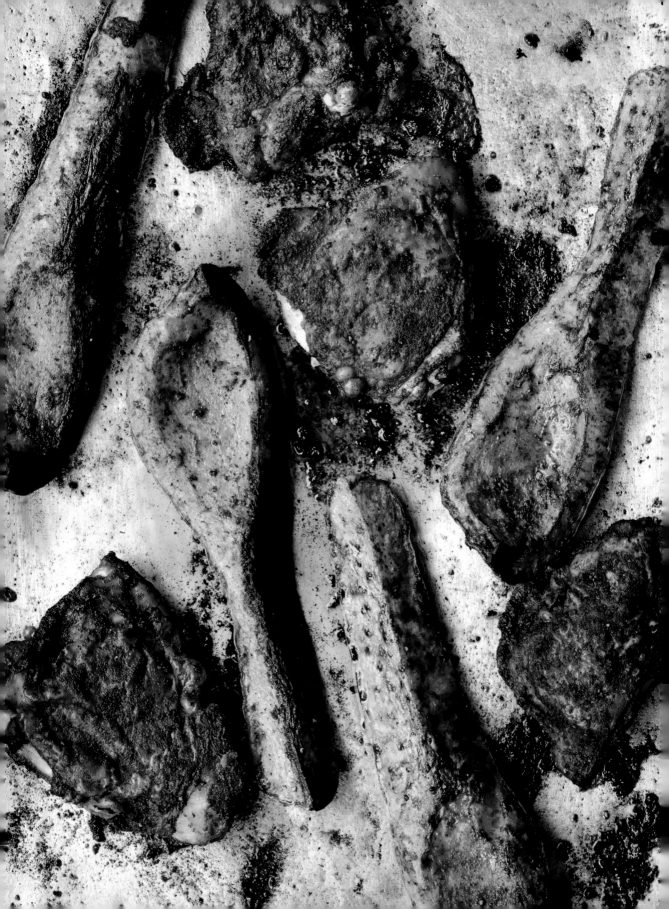

Sheet Pan Chicken Thighs and Butternut Squash

Serves 4

¼ cup **extra-virgin olive oil**

2 teaspoons **paprika**

1 teaspoon **ground cinnamon**

1 teaspoon **ground ginger**

1 teaspoon **cayenne pepper**

8 bone-in, skin-on **chicken thighs**

**Kosher salt and freshly ground
   black pepper**

1 small **butternut squash**, cut
   lengthwise and seeded

I'll admit that when everybody started going crazy about this whole "sheet-pan cooking" thing, I was a little amused. As a chef, the technique of throwing a bunch of stuff on a sheet tray and tossing it in the oven runs counter to everything I learned in culinary school, where we were taught to give each ingredient its own attention. Boy, was I wrong! You can really have fun with this method by experimenting with different ingredient and flavor combinations. The key is to pair foods that cook at the same speed. And the best part is, there's only one pan to clean up at the end! Serve this with Power Salad (page 109).

1. Preheat the oven to 425°F. Line 2 sheet pans with foil.

2. In a medium bowl, whisk together the olive oil, paprika, cinnamon, ginger, and cayenne.

3. Using paper towels, pat the chicken dry. Season both sides with a pinch of salt and a twist of black pepper. Coat both sides of the chicken with half of the spice paste and arrange skin-side down on one of the pans, making sure to leave space between the pieces. Coat the exposed flesh of the squash quarters with the remaining spice mixture and arrange skin-side down on the other pan, making sure to leave space between the pieces.

4. Transfer both pans to the oven and cook for 45 minutes, occasionally turning the squash to achieve even browning. After 45 minutes, flip the chicken. Continue cooking until the squash is deeply caramelized and soft, and the chicken is golden brown and the thickest part reaches an internal temperature of 160°F, about 15 minutes longer.

Rigatoni with Tomatoes, Eggplant, and Jalapeños

Serves 6

Kosher salt and freshly ground
 black pepper

1 pound **rigatoni**

¼ cup **extra-virgin olive oil**, plus
 more for drizzling

2 large **eggplants**, peeled and cut
 into ½-inch cubes (about 10 cups)

2 **garlic cloves**, thinly sliced

1 **jalapeño**, thinly sliced crosswise

1 pint **cherry tomatoes**, halved

2 cups **fresh basil leaves**

I grow eggplants in my garden and I'm always looking for great ways to prepare them other than baba ghanoush (which I love!). This recipe combines a bunch of garden staples, like tomatoes, hot peppers, and fragrant fresh basil into one wholesome Mediterranean-style pasta. The sautéed tomatoes and eggplant combined with the reserved pasta water create a silky, rich, and satisfying sauce that rivals those made with butter, cream, or parm (or all three).

1. Add 3 tablespoons salt to a large pot of water and bring to a boil over high heat. Add the pasta and cook until just al dente, about 1 minute less than the package directions. Occasionally give the pasta a stir so it doesn't stick together. Scoop out and reserve 1 cup of the pasta water before draining the pasta.

2. Meanwhile, place a large skillet over medium-high heat. Add the olive oil and heat to shimmering, then add the eggplant and a large pinch of salt. Stir to evenly coat the eggplant in oil. Cook, stirring occasionally, until the eggplant softens and begins to brown, about 10 minutes. Add the garlic and jalapeño and cook until aromatic, about 2 minutes. If the pan appears dry, add a splash of olive oil.

3. Reduce the heat to medium, add the tomatoes, and cook until they soften and break down, about 2 minutes. Add the drained pasta and reserved pasta water to the pan and cook for 30 seconds, stirring to blend. Season with salt and pepper to taste.

4. Remove the pan from the heat, stir in the basil leaves, finish with a good drizzle of olive oil, and serve.

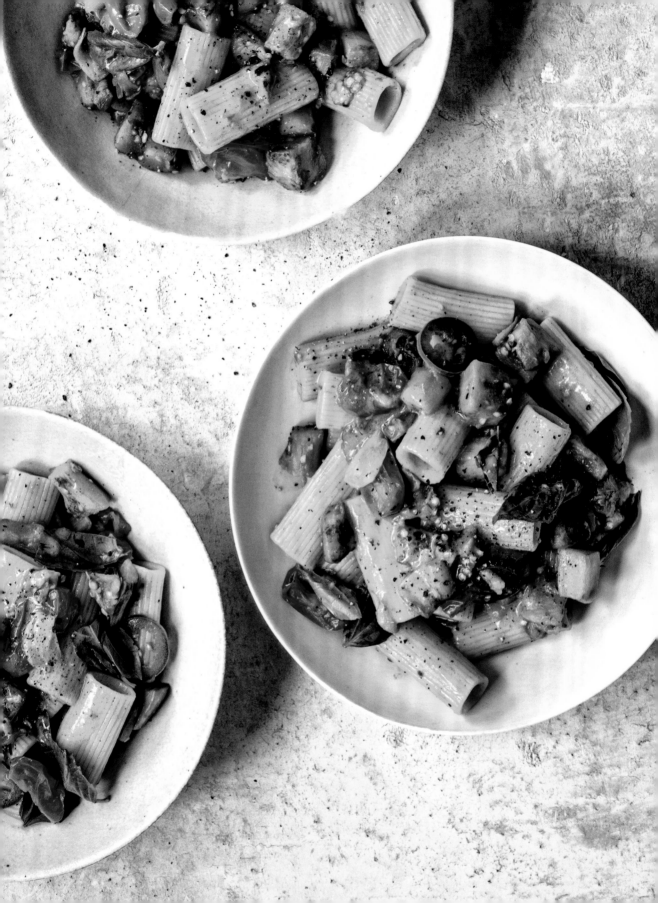

"Cheesy" Mashed Celery Root

Serves 6

4 cups **unsweetened oat milk**

2 medium **celery roots**, peeled and cut into 1-inch chunks

1 tablespoon **ground turmeric**

1 teaspoon **freshly grated nutmeg**

Kosher salt and freshly ground black pepper

4 medium **russet potatoes**, peeled and cut into 1-inch cubes

¾ cup **nutritional yeast**

Thanks to the magic of oat milk, a nondairy alternative to the real thing, I am able to enjoy starchy side dishes like this one that deliver on the comfort without bringing a world of hurt onto my joints. Unlike plain-old potatoes, celery root (also called celeriac) supplies tons of earthy flavor while delivering on the fiber, vitamin, and antioxidant fronts. The oat milk provides the creamy consistency. And the nutritional yeast gives the mash a satisfying cheese-like nuttiness. The turmeric is a great anti-inflammatory bonus, so I add it to the party.

1. In a large saucepan, combine the oat milk, celery root, turmeric, nutmeg, a large pinch of salt, and ¼ teaspoon black pepper and bring to a gentle simmer over medium-high heat. Cook until the celery root is easily pierced with a knife, about 25 minutes. Scoop out and reserve 1½ cups of the cooking liquid before draining.

2. Transfer the celery root to a large bowl and press with a potato masher until smooth. Set aside.

3. Place the potatoes in the saucepan, cover with cold water by a few inches, add a large pinch of salt, and bring to a boil over medium-high heat. Cook, partially covered, until the potatoes are easily pierced with a knife, about 15 minutes. Drain, return the potatoes to the pan, and press with a potato masher until smooth.

4. Return the mashed celery root to the pan with the mashed potatoes and add 1 cup of the reserved cooking liquid and the nutritional yeast. Stir to combine and season with a pinch of salt and a twist of black pepper. If the mixture appears a little dry, stir in the remaining cooking liquid. Serve warm.

Roasted Carrots

with Cumin and Cinnamon

Serves 6

2 pounds **carrots** (preferably organic), with tops

¼ cup **extra-virgin olive oil**

2 tablespoons **raw honey**

2 tablespoons **cumin seeds**

1 teaspoon **ground cinnamon**

1 teaspoon **paprika**

Kosher salt and freshly ground black pepper

Grated zest and juice of 1 orange

Flaky sea salt, such as Maldon, for finishing

Roasting brings out the natural sweetness in carrots. When set against the warm spices of cumin and cinnamon, you end up with a really special, but very simple, autumn side dish. To get the most nutrients out of this, I use whole unpeeled organic bunch carrots, because it's been proven that the peel and the flesh just below it are loaded with vitamins A, K, and biotin, a B vitamin. Just make sure that they are well cleaned. If you don't go organic, then peel and scrub to get rid of those potential pesticides.

1. Preheat the oven to 425°F. Line a sheet pan with parchment paper.

2. Remove the carrot tops, roughly chop, and set aside. Scrub but do not peel the carrots.

3. In a large bowl, whisk together the olive oil, honey, cumin seeds, cinnamon, and paprika. Add the carrots and toss to coat with the honey mixture.

4. Arrange the carrots in a single layer on the prepared sheet pan, making sure to leave some space between them. Season with a pinch of salt and a twist of black pepper and cook for 10 minutes. Turn the carrots and cook until they are slightly tender, but still have a little bite, about 10 minutes more.

5. Transfer the carrots to a serving platter and top with the orange zest and juice, any accumulated juices from the sheet pan, and the chopped carrot tops. Garnish with flaky sea salt and serve.

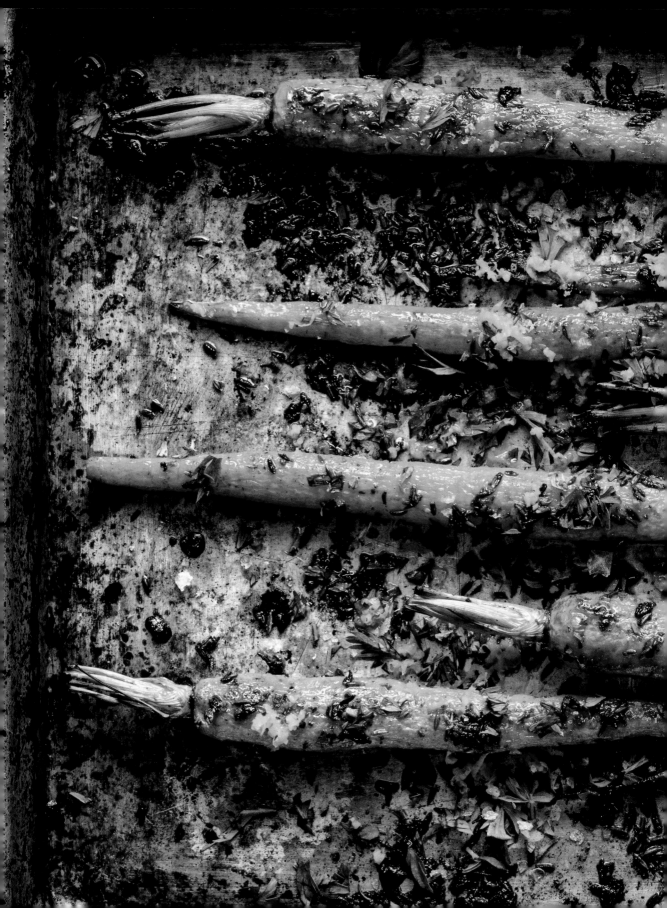

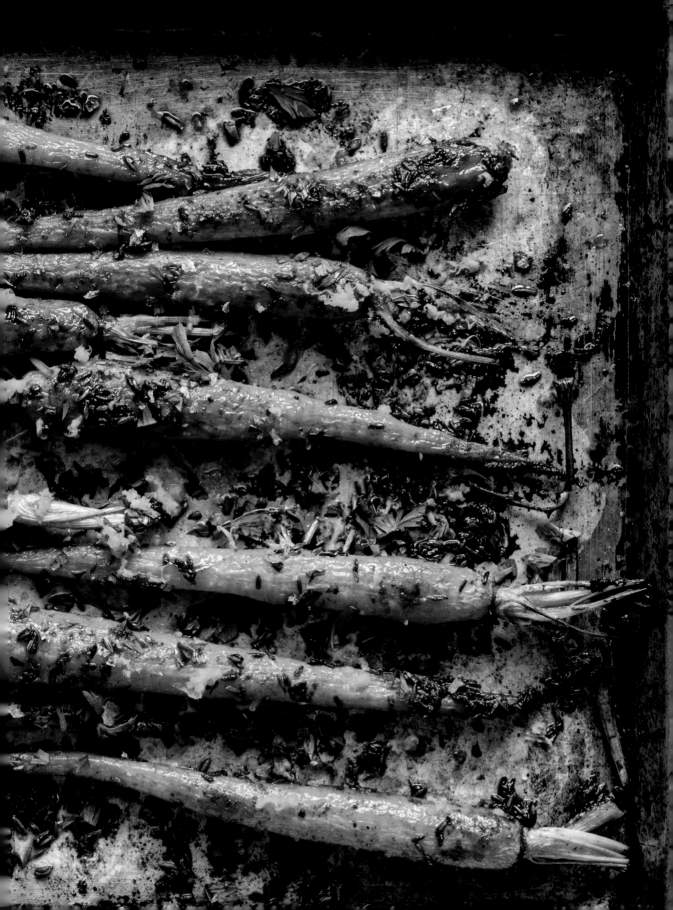

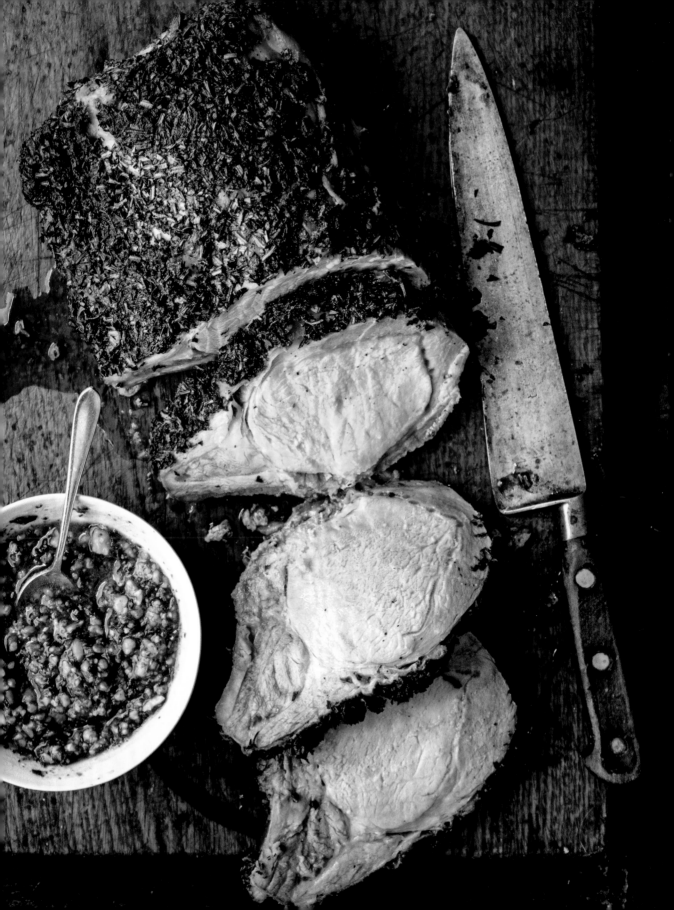

Roasted Rack of Pork

with Crushed Walnut Sauce

Serves 4

1 (4-bone) **pork rib roast** (about 2½ pounds)

1 cup **walnut halves**

1 tablespoon finely chopped **fresh rosemary**

1 tablespoon finely chopped **fresh oregano**

1 tablespoon finely chopped **fresh flat-leaf parsley**

2 tablespoons **Dijon mustard**

Kosher salt and freshly ground black pepper

½ cup **extra-virgin olive oil**

Juice of ½ lemon

1 cup **spinach leaves**

1 **garlic clove**, minced

This is an impressive Sunday supper if ever there was one. Sometimes called a pork rib roast, this cut is generously marbled with fat so it stays juicy, and the bones add a ton of flavor. The roast ends up with a great crust from the mustard and herb rub, and the lemony walnut sauce helps to cut through the richness. Pork and fruit go hand in hand, so consider serving this with the Miso and Tamari–Roasted Pears with Pomegranate (page 114).

1. Preheat the oven to 350°F.

2. Take the pork from the refrigerator, remove the packaging, set it on a large plate or platter, and allow it to come to room temperature, about 45 minutes.

3. Place the walnuts on a sheet pan and cook until aromatic and lightly toasted, about 8 minutes. Transfer to a bowl or plate and set aside.

4. Increase the oven temperature to 400°F.

5. In a medium bowl, mix together the rosemary, oregano, and parsley. Using paper towels, pat the pork dry. Coat the meat on all sides with the mustard, season liberally with salt and pepper, and evenly distribute and press the herb mixture over the ends and sides of the pork.

6. Place the pork on a wire rack set onto a sheet pan and cook until the thickest part of the roast reaches an internal temperature of 145°F, about 1 hour. Remove the pork from the oven and transfer it to a cutting board. Set aside to rest, loosely tented with foil, for 20 minutes.

7. Meanwhile, in a blender or food processor, combine the toasted walnuts, olive oil, lemon juice, spinach, and garlic and pulse until chunky, about 10 times. Taste and add salt and pepper if needed.

8. To serve, slice the pork between the bones into chops and top with walnut sauce.

Dairy-Free Fix

Farro Salad

with Pine Nuts, Peaches, Blueberries, and Spinach

Serves 6

1½ cups **dried farro**

¼ cup **pine nuts**

½ cup **orange juice**, preferably freshly squeezed

Kosher salt and freshly ground black pepper

½ cup **extra-virgin olive oil**

¼ cup **sherry vinegar**

2 teaspoons **raw honey**

2 **peaches**, halved, pitted, and thinly sliced

1 cup **blueberries**

2 cups roughly torn **baby spinach**

1 cup roughly torn **fresh basil leaves**

Ever since trying something similar at the restaurant Charlie Bird in New York, Liz has been on a farro salad kick. There's no need for cheese when you can squeeze so much flavor from high-nutrient additions like blueberries, spinach, and farro. Feel free to mix and match the fruits, greens, and nuts based on what's in season and what's on hand. You pretty much can't go wrong! This salad is best enjoyed freshly made.

1. Place the farro in a medium bowl, cover with cool water, and let soak for 20 minutes. Drain and set aside.

2. Preheat the oven to 350°F.

3. Place the pine nuts on a sheet pan and cook until lightly toasted, about 6 minutes. Set aside.

4. In a medium saucepan, combine 3 cups water, the orange juice, drained farro, and a pinch of salt. Bring to a boil over high heat, then reduce the heat to low to maintain a gentle simmer. Cook, partially covered, until the farro is tender, about 15 minutes. Drain the farro and set aside to cool.

5. Meanwhile, in a large bowl, whisk together the olive oil, vinegar, and honey. Season with a pinch of salt and a twist of black pepper.

6. Add the cooled farro, the peaches, blueberries, spinach, and basil to the dressing and toss together. Taste and add salt and pepper if needed. Serve at room temperature.

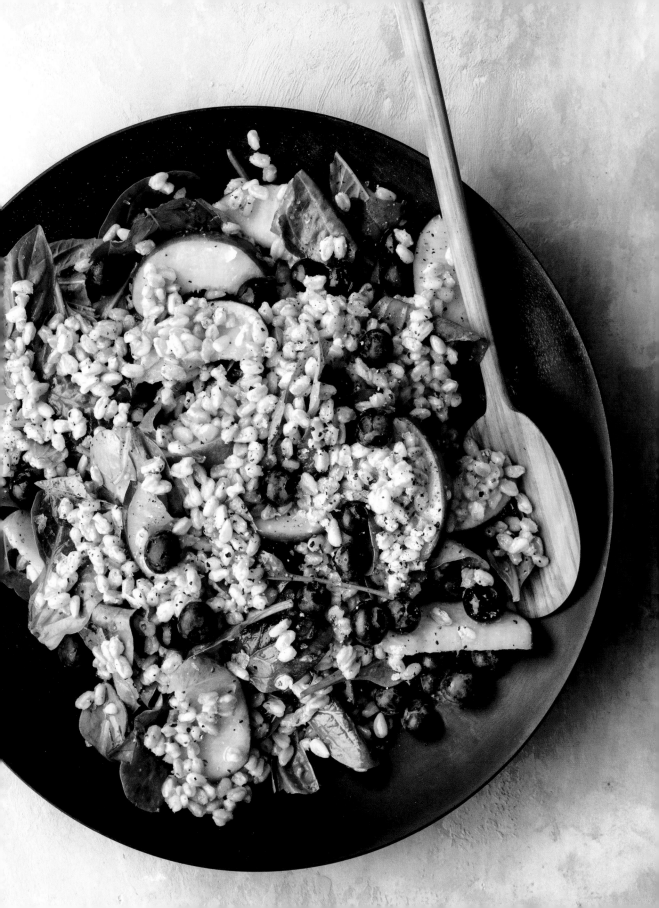

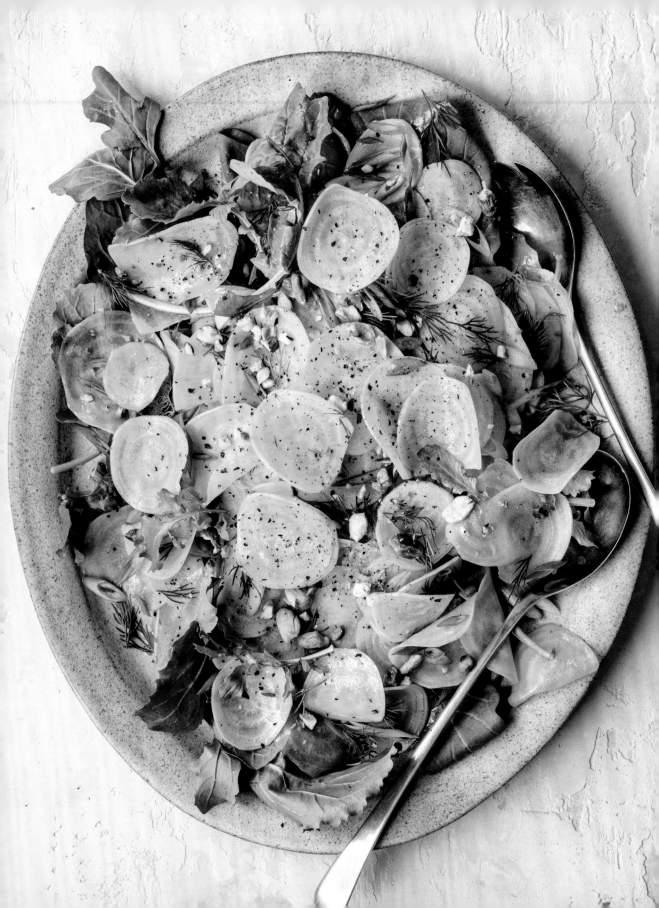

Shaved Beet Salad

Serves 6

¼ cup **extra-virgin olive oil**

2 tablespoons **sherry vinegar**

1 teaspoon **Dijon mustard**

¼ cup finely chopped **fresh dill**

Kosher salt and freshly ground black pepper

2 pounds **golden beets**, peeled and sliced ⅛ inch thick (using a chef's knife or mandoline)

4 cups **baby arugula**

1 cup thinly sliced **scallions**

½ cup chopped **roasted salted pistachios**

If you have any of my other cookbooks, then you know that I love beets. I enjoy them raw, roasted, smoked, and pickled. That said, I know that beets can be a divisive vegetable. If you *think* that you don't like beets, give this recipe a try, because it's light, crunchy, and accented with fresh, summery dill. When shopping, look for golden or candy-striped varieties, which have a milder flavor. As an added bonus, they won't stain your hands blood-red! I recommend using a mandoline or vegetable slicer to cut the beets super-thin, but a really sharp knife and steady hand works, too.

1. In a large bowl, whisk together the olive oil, vinegar, mustard, and dill. Season with a pinch of salt and a twist of black pepper.

2. Add the beets, arugula, scallions, and pistachios and toss well to combine. Taste and adjust for seasoning, adding salt and pepper as needed.

Kyle's Coconut Rice

Serves 6

2 tablespoons **coconut oil**

1 small **yellow onion**, finely chopped

2 **garlic cloves**, minced

2 tablespoons grated **fresh ginger**

1 **jalapeño**, seeded and finely chopped

Kosher salt and freshly ground black pepper

2 cups **basmati rice**, rinsed and drained

½ cup **unsweetened shredded coconut**

3 cups **chicken stock**, homemade or good-quality store-bought

1 cup **unsweetened full-fat coconut milk**

1 teaspoon **freshly grated nutmeg**

Grated zest of 1 lime

1 cup thinly sliced **scallions**

I take no credit for this recipe as it is 100 percent Liz, who has been making a version of it for Kyle since he was little. If you're craving something creamy and starchy, but are looking for brighter, more tropical flavors, this is the dish. There really isn't any food that it doesn't go great with, from roasted vegetables and grilled fish to long-braised meats.

1. Place a large saucepan over medium heat. Add the coconut oil and heat to shimmering, then add the onion, garlic, ginger, jalapeño, and a pinch of salt and cook until the vegetables are aromatic and soft, stirring occasionally, about 3 minutes. Add the rice and shredded coconut and cook until very fragrant, stirring occasionally, about 3 minutes.

2. Stir in the chicken stock, coconut milk, and nutmeg and season with a pinch of salt and a twist of black pepper. Bring to a boil, then reduce the heat to low to maintain a gentle simmer. Cover and cook until the rice is tender and the liquid is absorbed, about 18 minutes.

3. Remove the pan from the heat and sprinkle on the lime zest and scallions. Fluff and toss with a fork and serve.

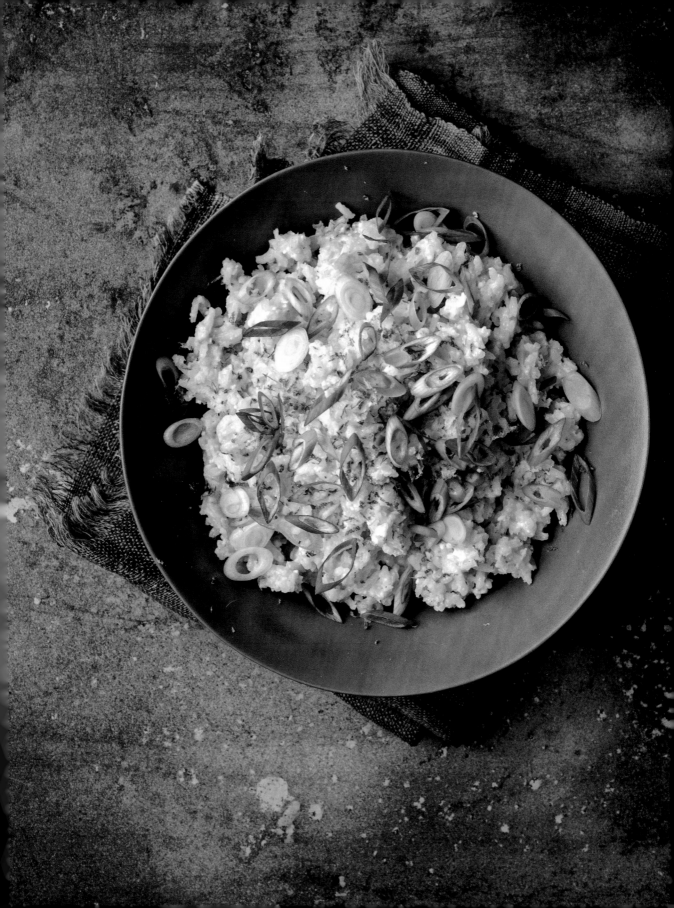

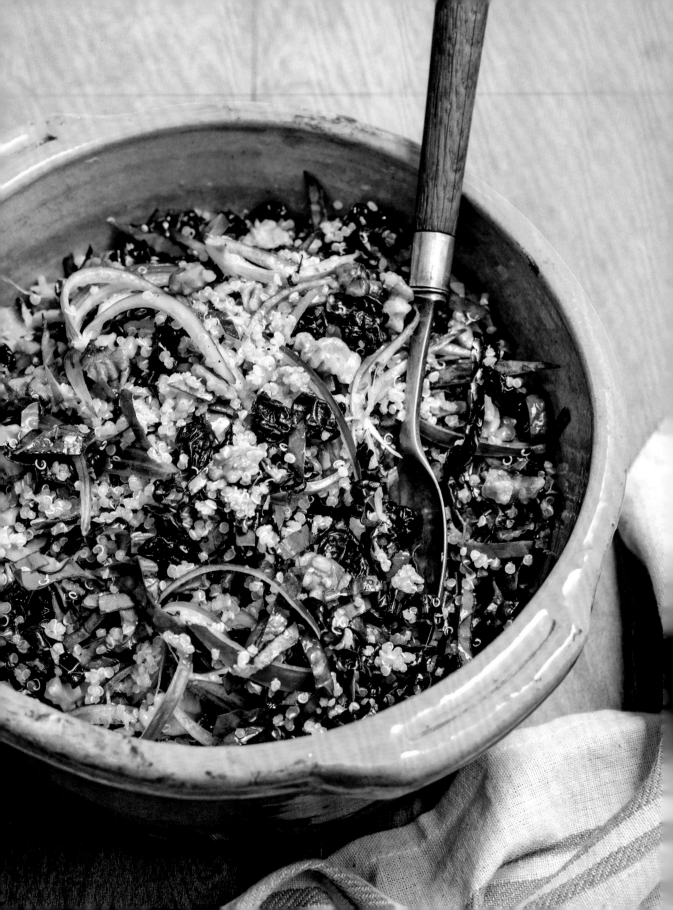

Power Salad

Serves 6

½ cup **walnut halves**

1 cup **quinoa**, rinsed

Kosher salt and freshly ground black pepper

½ cup **dried cherries**

½ cup **extra-virgin olive oil**

¼ cup **red wine vinegar**

1 teaspoon **Dijon mustard**

1 teaspoon **raw honey**

1 small **red onion**, halved and thinly sliced

3 cups finely sliced **kale leaves and tender stems**

3 cups finely sliced **baby spinach**

1 **garlic clove**, minced

The name is no exaggeration: This salad is like high-test fuel for your body thanks to the leafy greens, nutrient-rich quinoa, and energy-packed dried fruit. Whenever I feel a little run down or am staring down a huge day, I'll dig into a deep bowl of this superfood. Loaded with nuts, dried fruit, seeds, and honey (without a trace of cheese!), it's essentially the salad version of granola. It's perfect on its own or as a side dish to Grilled Skirt Steak with Cherry-Balsamic Sauce (page 90).

1. Preheat the oven to 350°F.

2. Arrange the walnuts on a sheet pan and cook until aromatic and lightly toasted, about 8 minutes. Set aside.

3. In a medium saucepan, combine 2 cups water, the quinoa, and a pinch of salt. Bring to a boil over high heat and then reduce the heat to low to maintain a gentle simmer. Cook, partially covered, until the quinoa pops open and becomes tender, about 15 minutes. Remove from the heat, sprinkle the dried cherries on top of the quinoa, cover, and set aside while you make the vinaigrette.

4. Meanwhile, in a large bowl, whisk together the olive oil, vinegar, mustard, and honey. Season with a pinch of salt and a twist of black pepper. Add the onion, toss to combine, and set aside for 5 minutes.

5. Add the quinoa, kale, spinach, and garlic to the dressing and toss to combine. Taste and adjust for seasoning, adding salt and pepper as needed.

Blackberry, Almond, and Goji Salad

Serves 6

⅓ cup slivered **almonds**

½ cup **extra-virgin olive oil**

¼ cup **red wine vinegar**

1 small **red onion**, halved and thinly sliced

¼ cup **dried goji berries**

2 cups **blackberries**

⅓ cup torn **fresh mint leaves**

Kosher salt and freshly ground black pepper

This salad is a powerhouse of vitamins and minerals thanks to antioxidant-rich blackberries and goji berries, which are easier than ever to find and boost immunity while also fighting inflammation. In the summer, when the mint patch and berry bushes are going crazy, I will make this crunch-filled salad—or a version of it—every other day.

1. Preheat the oven to 350°F.

2. Place the almonds on a sheet pan and cook until lightly toasted, about 8 minutes. Set aside.

3. In a large bowl, whisk together the olive oil and vinegar. Add the onion and goji berries, toss together, and set aside for 10 minutes.

4. Add the blackberries, mint, and toasted almonds to the vinaigrette and gently toss together. Taste and adjust for seasoning, adding salt and pepper as needed.

Roasted Pineapple and Pepper Salad

Serves 6

1 **pineapple**, peeled, quartered lengthwise, and core sliced away

¼ cup **extra-virgin olive oil**, plus more for roasting

Kosher salt and freshly ground black pepper

Grated zest and juice of 2 limes

½ teaspoon **ground turmeric**

1 fresh **Fresno chile**, thinly sliced crosswise

1 **red bell pepper**, halved and thinly sliced

½ cup roughly chopped **fresh cilantro leaves**

½ cup thinly sliced **scallions**

There are two types of people in the world: those who like pineapple on their pizza and those with good taste. I'm firmly in the second camp, but that doesn't mean that I don't love cooked pineapple. This tropical fruit is a great source of bromelain, which is good at reducing inflammation. Roasting the fruit intensifies its natural sweetness while enhancing the tropical flavors. When cooled, the juicy-ripe fruit makes the perfect base for all kinds of sweet and savory salads. This one would go great with grilled seafood or Grilled Chicken Paillard (page 85) but maybe not pizza.

1. Preheat the oven to 500°F.

2. Coat all sides of the pineapple with some olive oil, season with a pinch of salt and a twist of black pepper, arrange in a single layer on a sheet pan, and cook until beginning to char, about 10 minutes. Turn the pineapple and continue cooking until charred and beginning to soften, about 10 minutes longer. When cool enough to handle, cut the roasted pineapple into ¼-inch dice and set aside.

3. Meanwhile, in a large bowl, whisk together the ¼ cup olive oil, lime zest, lime juice, turmeric, Fresno chile, and ½ teaspoon black pepper. Season with salt.

4. Add the pineapple, bell pepper, cilantro, and scallions to the dressing and toss together. Taste and adjust for seasoning, adding salt and pepper as needed.

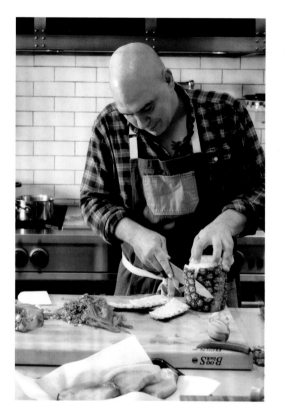

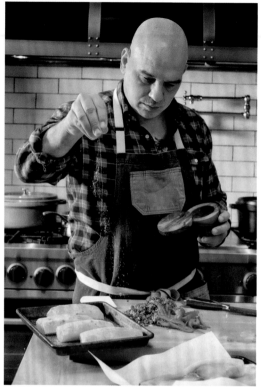

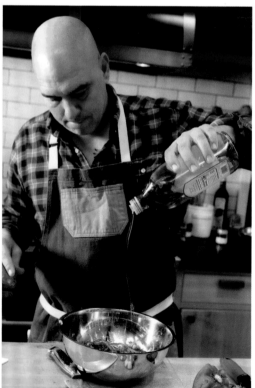

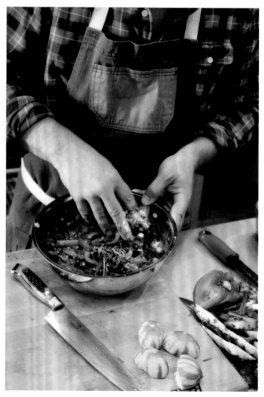

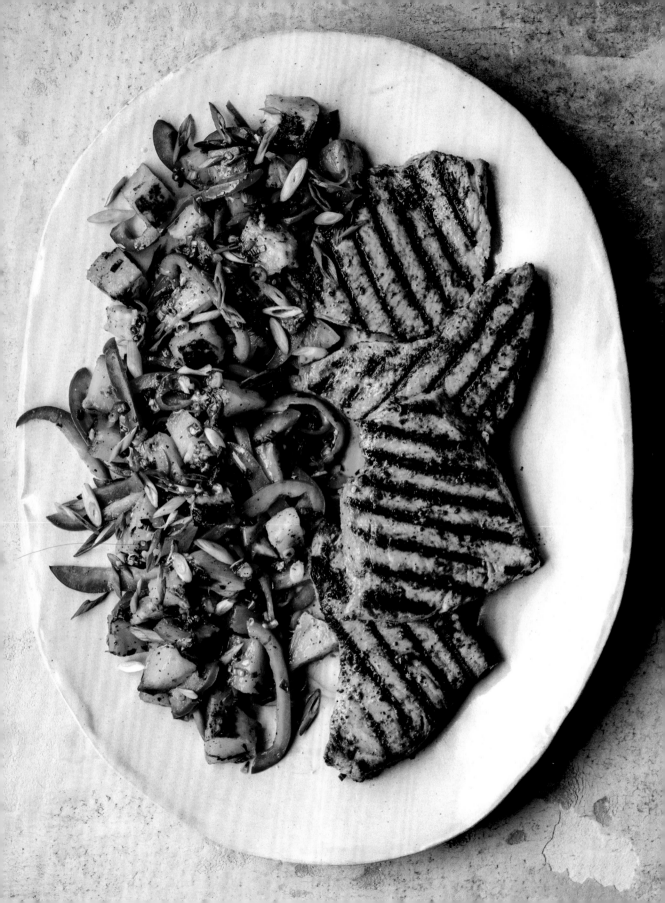

Miso and Tamari-Roasted Pears

with Pomegranate

Serves 6

3 tablespoons **rice vinegar**

2 tablespoons **tamari** (wheat-free soy sauce)

2 tablespoons **white miso**

2 tablespoons **pure maple syrup**

½ teaspoon **ground ginger**

¼ teaspoon **cayenne pepper**

4 ripe **pears** (I like Bartlett), peeled, halved, and cored

⅓ cup **pomegranate seeds**

Roasting (or grilling) fruit amplifies its natural sweetness. When contrasted with a savory soy and miso glaze, you end up with something unique and captivating. In fall, when pears are ripe, flavorful, and plentiful, I love to serve this with meat dishes like Roasted Rack of Pork with Crushed Walnut Sauce (page 101). The leftover pears also make a great breakfast when topped with a few scoops of homemade Coconut-Cashew Granola (page 235).

1. Preheat the oven to 450°F. Line a sheet pan with foil.

2. In a medium bowl, whisk together the vinegar, tamari, miso, maple syrup, ginger, and cayenne. Evenly coat the pears in half of this mixture and place them, cut-side down, on the lined sheet pan. Set aside the remaining sauce.

3. Roast the pears until they begin to caramelize and soften, about 10 minutes. Increase the oven temperature to 500°F, flip the pears, and divide the remaining sauce into the hollows of each one. Continue cooking until sticky and deeply caramelized, about 12 minutes.

4. Top with pomegranate seeds and serve.

Warm Baby Kale and Mushroom Salad

Serves 4

2 large **eggs**

6 tablespoons **extra-virgin olive oil**, plus more for cooking

¼ cup **red wine vinegar**

2 teaspoons **Dijon mustard**

Kosher salt and freshly ground black pepper

6 cups sliced **wild mushrooms** (such as cremini and maitake), tough stems removed

1 small **red onion**, finely chopped

1 **garlic clove**, minced

1 tablespoon finely chopped **fresh thyme leaves**

10 ounces **baby kale**

½ cup **dried goji berries** (optional)

I grew up eating a version of this salad, but it was made with spinach and raw button mushrooms and the dressing was cloyingly sweet. This is a grown-up edition starring sautéed wild mushrooms and a classic vinaigrette. Thanks to the cooked eggs and heaps of baby kale, this nutritious salad makes an ideal lunch.

1. Place the eggs in a small saucepan, cover with cold water and bring to a boil over high heat. Once boiling, turn off the heat and let the eggs sit, covered, for 11 minutes. Meanwhile, fill a medium bowl with ice and water. Drain and then shock them in the ice bath. Peel, slice, and set aside.

2. In a small bowl, whisk together the olive oil, vinegar, and mustard. Season with a pinch of salt and a twist of black pepper; set aside.

3. Place a large heavy-bottomed skillet over high heat. Add a drizzle of olive oil and heat to shimmering, then add the mushrooms. Cook, stirring occasionally, until they have given up most of their liquid and begun to brown, about 5 minutes. If the mushrooms don't all fit at once, cook them in batches (otherwise, they will steam instead of brown). Transfer the mushrooms to a plate and set aside.

4. Set the skillet back over medium heat, coat the pan with a drizzle of olive oil, and add the onion, garlic, thyme, and pinch of salt. Cook until the vegetables are aromatic and softened, stirring occasionally, about 3 minutes. Return the mushrooms to the pan and season with another pinch of salt and pepper. Remove the pan from the heat, add half of the vinaigrette, and use a wooden spoon to stir and loosen any browned bits on the bottom of the pan.

5. In a large bowl, combine the kale, sliced eggs, goji berries (if using), and mushroom mixture and toss together. Taste and adjust for seasoning, adding more vinaigrette, salt, and pepper as needed.

Dairy-Free Fix

Flour-Free Fix

Like some people, after eating flour-based foods such as bagels, breads, pastas, and crackers, I'd feel lousy. I quickly jumped to the conclusion that the reason was because I had a sensitivity to wheat and gluten. After lots of experimentation, however, I discovered that it wasn't *all* flour that was triggering my flare-ups, but rather the type of flour that I was consuming.

My moment of reckoning dawned on me after I returned from a trip to Italy, where I ate pasta every single day. Unlike when I ate pasta in the States, I experienced zero discomfort. I began to think that there was more to this flour debate than meets the stomach. Some of my favorite bakeries and restaurants, in New York and beyond, mill their own organic grains fresh every day. I noticed that after eating rolls, buns, and baguettes made with these old-fashioned, freshly ground, whole-grain flours, I had zero problems with flare-ups and pain. The real turning point was when my stepson, Kyle, was preparing to open Grindstone, his doughnut shop in Sag Harbor, New York. Kyle originally was determined to mill his own local flour and, given my topsy-turvy history with flour, I was interested in helping him do the research. What I learned was fascinating.

Over the past few decades, the way we farm and process wheat has changed so dramatically that today's flour barely resembles the stuff that our parents and grandparents baked with. From hybridized and genetically modified seeds to chemical fertilizers and pesticides, farmers are going to extreme lengths to increase yield and maximize production. Modern milling practices remove the germ and bran from the grain to make white "all-purpose" flour, stripping out most of the beneficial vitamins and minerals to make a product that's cheaper, more shelf-stable, and more easily produced. The resulting fluff is often bleached to a snow-white color, bromated to improve baking, and then enriched to add back all the nutrients that were removed earlier in the process, while still lacking in benefits that whole wheat originally brought to the table. The truth is, many of these additives and processes are illegal outside of the United States for good reason. Potassium bromate, for example, is an oxidizing agent that can be dangerous when not fully depleted during the baking process.

Now, I'm not saying that someone who suffers from celiac disease can just switch to good-quality flour and be fine. For the estimated 1 percent of people who have that condition, the ingestion of gluten is a dangerous and painful event. What I'm talking about is the far less serious issue of wheat sensitivity, which is completely different. For those people, I do think that by switching to products made with organic whole-grain, stone-milled flour, much of the discomfort would disappear. Regardless, this chapter foregoes flour altogether because it remains a trigger for so many people.

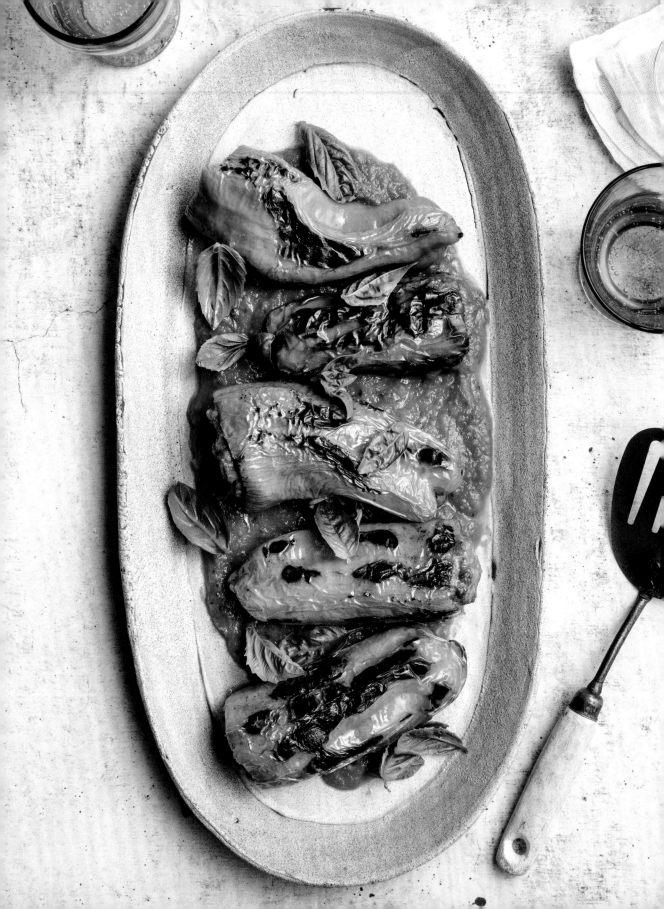

Sausage-Stuffed Hot Peppers

Serves 4 to 8

I got my green thumb from my grandfather, who grew amazing hot peppers in his vegetable garden. One of my favorite ways to eat them was when they were stuffed with zesty Italian sausage and served with *pomodoro* sauce—no bread crumbs needed. Eating them was a little like playing Russian roulette—you never knew when you'd get a crazy spicy pepper! If you can't find Hungarian hot (or wax) peppers, which are large, sweet, and mild, you can substitute equally tame Anaheim peppers.

Extra-virgin olive oil

2 cups **Pomodoro Sauce** (page 131) or store-bought marinara sauce

8 **Hungarian hot peppers**

1½ pounds **sweet Italian sausage**, removed from the casings if not bulk

½ cup torn **fresh basil leaves**

1. Preheat the oven to 375°F.

2. Grease an 8 × 11-inch baking dish with olive oil, spread the pomodoro sauce evenly over the bottom, and set aside.

3. Remove the stem ends of the peppers and spoon out the seeds, being careful to keep the peppers intact. Divide the sausage equally among the peppers, loosely stuffing them to the top.

4. Preheat a grill or grill pan to medium-high heat.

5. Drizzle some olive oil over the peppers and place them on the grill. Cook until nicely charred, about 2 minutes, flip, and continue cooking until the other side is nicely charred, about 2 minutes more. Arrange the peppers on top of the pomodoro sauce.

6. Bake the peppers in the oven until the sausage reaches an internal temperature of 160°F, about 10 minutes. Transfer them to a platter, top with pomodoro sauce from the pan, and garnish with fresh basil.

Zucchini Noodles

with Corn, Tomatoes, Dill, and Feta

Serves 4

4 medium **zucchini** or 2 pounds zucchini noodles/zoodles

½ cup **extra-virgin olive oil**

2 **garlic cloves**, minced

Kosher salt and freshly ground black pepper

2 cups **fresh corn kernels**

2 cups halved **cherry tomatoes**

½ cup finely chopped **fresh dill**

½ cup crumbled **feta cheese**

When you love to garden like I do, half the fun is coming up with delicious ways to utilize all of the fresh bounty. This is one of my favorite recipes in peak summer, when almost everything I need is just steps from my kitchen door. Don't leave out the dill; I think it really makes the entire dish. If you don't have a vegetable spiralizer (a cool tool that turns vegetables into long ribbons), look for an affordable julienne peeler, which works almost as well. These days, many groceries sell bagged "zoodles," sometimes labeled as veggie spirals or zucchini noodles.

1. Use a vegetable spiralizer or julienne peeler to cut the zucchini into long noodles. If you don't have either of those kitchen tools, cut each zucchini lengthwise into ⅛-inch-thick slices and then cut the slices lengthwise into thin, long strands.

2. Set a large skillet over low heat. Add the olive oil, followed by the garlic and a pinch of salt. Cook until the garlic is fragrant, about 1 minute. Increase the heat to medium, add the zucchini noodles and corn, and season with a pinch of salt and a twist of black pepper. Cook, stirring to combine, until the zucchini begins to soften, about 3 minutes.

3. Add the tomatoes and continue cooking until the vegetables are very tender, about 3 minutes more. Remove from the heat, top with the dill and feta, and serve.

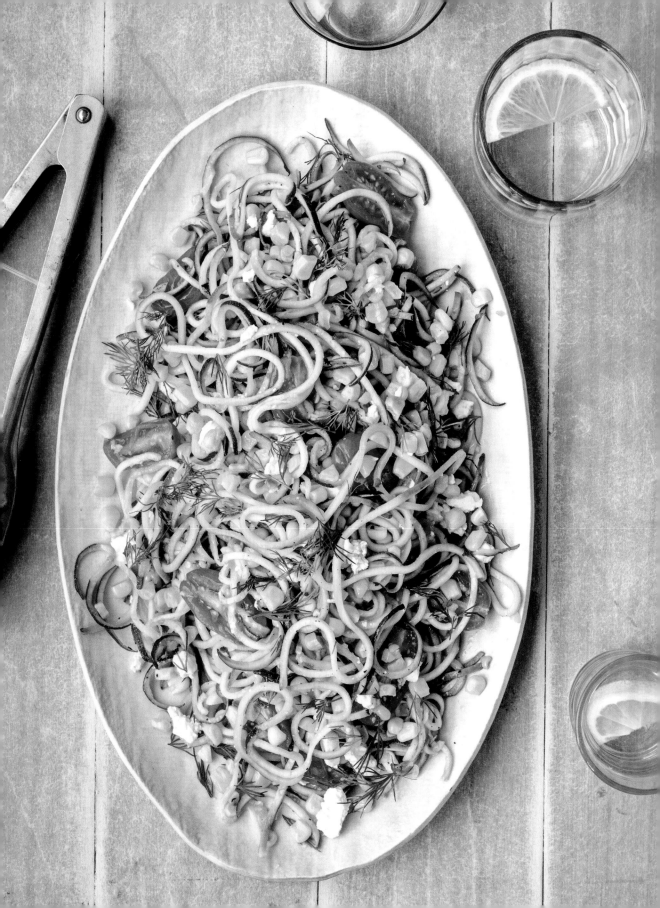

Mushroom and Cauliflower "Risotto"

This cauliflower-based risotto is much lighter than the traditional versions that call for Arborio rice, but it's every bit as flavorful. If you want to make it with rice, you can—it will be just as tasty, though you might have to tinker with the amount of liquid used. This dish is great as a side dish or as a vegetarian main course.

Serves 6

2 tablespoons **extra-virgin olive oil**

5 tablespoons **unsalted butter**

3 cups **cremini mushrooms**, tough stems removed, finely chopped

1 small **yellow onion**, finely chopped

2 **garlic cloves**, minced

Kosher salt and freshly ground black pepper

2 tablespoons **fresh thyme leaves**, finely chopped

1 small head **cauliflower**, cut into small florets

¼ cup **dry white wine**

1 cup **Vegetable Stock**, homemade (page 240) or good-quality store-bought

⅔ cup **freshly grated parmesan cheese**

1. Set a large heavy-bottomed skillet over medium-high heat. Add the olive oil and 2 tablespoons of the butter and heat until the butter is melted, then add the mushrooms. Cook until the mushrooms have given up most of their liquid and begun to brown, about 3 minutes. Add the onion, garlic, and a pinch of salt and continue cooking until the vegetables begin to soften, about 3 minutes. Stir in the thyme and cauliflower and continue cooking until the cauliflower begins to soften, about 2 minutes.

2. Add the wine and cook, stirring constantly, until most of the liquid has evaporated, about 2 minutes. Add the stock and cook, stirring constantly, until most of the liquid has evaporated, about 5 minutes.

3. Remove from the heat, add the remaining 3 tablespoons butter and the parmesan, stir to combine, and serve.

Loaded Greens

with Walnuts and Mushrooms

Serves 4

3 tablespoons **extra-virgin olive oil**, plus more if needed

1 small **yellow onion**, thinly sliced

3 cups thinly sliced **cremini mushrooms**, tough stems removed

Kosher salt and freshly ground black pepper

1 cup **walnut halves**, roughly chopped

2 pounds **collard greens**, stems removed and leaves roughly chopped

1 teaspoon **ground turmeric**

2 tablespoons **red wine vinegar**

I normally toss a meaty smoked ham hock into every pot of collard greens that I make, but this recipe goes in a slightly different direction. Thanks to the walnuts and mushrooms, which provide tons of depth and umami, I almost don't even miss the hock. Almost!

1. Place a large Dutch oven over medium heat. Add the olive oil and heat to shimmering, then add the onion, mushrooms, and a pinch of salt. Cook until the mushrooms have given up most of their liquid and begun to brown, about 5 minutes.

2. Add the walnuts and cook until toasted and fragrant, about 3 minutes. Add the collard greens in batches, stirring and waiting until they wilt, then add the next handful, until it all fits in the pan. Stir in the turmeric, ½ teaspoon black pepper, and a pinch of salt.

3. Reduce the heat to low, cover, and cook until completely wilted, about 5 minutes. Give the pot a stir, cover, and continue cooking, stirring occasionally, until the greens have softened, about 20 minutes.

4. Remove from the heat, stir in the vinegar, taste, and adjust for seasoning, adding salt and pepper as needed.

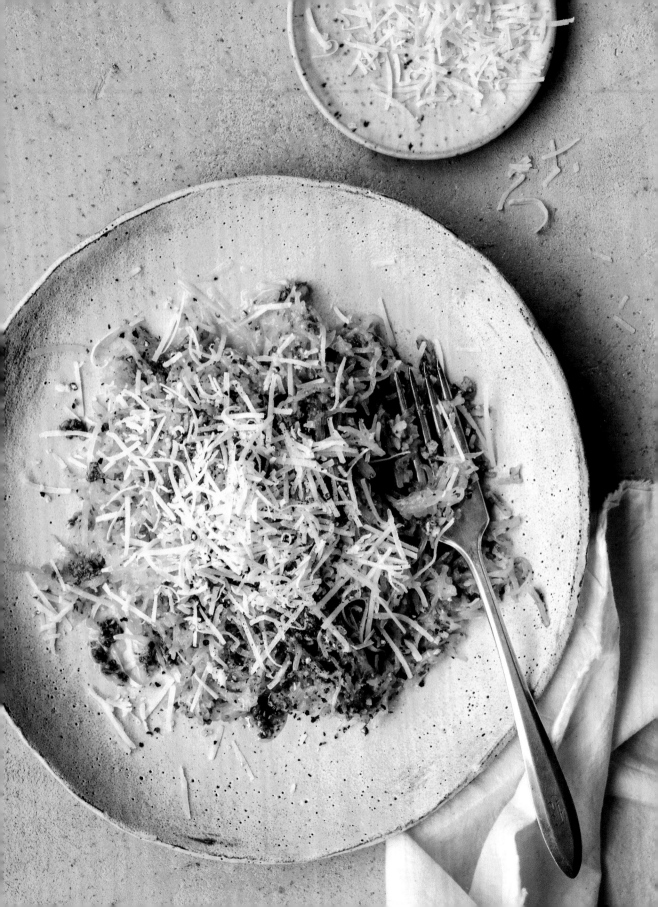

Spaghetti Squash

with Arugula Pesto

Serves 6

1 large **spaghetti squash**, halved lengthwise, seeds removed, cleaned, and rinsed

½ cup **extra-virgin olive oil**, plus more for cooking

Kosher salt and freshly ground black pepper

2 cups **arugula**

2 cups **fresh basil leaves**

2 **garlic cloves**, roughly chopped

½ cup **freshly grated parmesan cheese**

Juice of ½ lemon

Around the time that hardy squashes like butternut, acorn, and spaghetti begin to show up in the fall, my basil and arugula plants are on their way out. That's the perfect time to make a big batch of pesto, which goes great on long strands of pulled, roasted spaghetti squash. In place of expensive pine nuts, this pesto uses the seeds that come free with the squash! If, after removing the seeds from the squash, you don't end up with ⅓ cup, supplement with hulled pumpkin seeds, pine nuts, or another roasted nut.

1. Preheat the oven to 350°F. Line a sheet pan with foil.

2. Arrange the squash seeds in a single layer on the prepared sheet pan. Drizzle with 2 teaspoons olive oil and cook until they are lightly toasted and crisp, about 12 minutes. Transfer them to a plate and set aside (save the pan to roast the squash).

3. Increase the oven temperature to 400°F. Lightly coat the cut side of the squash with olive oil, season with a pinch of salt and a twist of black pepper, and place it cut-side down on the reserved sheet pan. Roast until tender, about 45 minutes. Carefully add ¼ cup water to the sheet pan and continue cooking until the squash is easily pierced with a paring knife, about 15 minutes. Remove the pan from the oven and set aside.

4. Meanwhile, in a blender or food processor, add the toasted squash seeds, arugula, basil, and garlic. Pulse until it has the texture of fine bread crumbs, about 5 times. Add the ½ cup olive oil and process until smooth. Add the parmesan and lemon juice and pulse until combined, about 3 times. Season with a pinch of salt and a twist of black pepper.

5. While still warm, use a fork to scrape the squash flesh into spaghetti-like strands. In a large bowl, toss together the squash, arugula pesto, and any accumulated juices from the sheet pan. Season with a pinch of salt and a twist of black pepper and serve.

Flour-Free Fix

125

Skillet Kale Gratin

Serves 6

1 tablespoon **extra-virgin olive oil**

1 large **yellow onion**, cut into ¼-inch dice

3 **garlic cloves**, minced

Kosher salt and freshly ground black pepper

3 pounds **kale leaves and tender stems**, sliced 1 inch thick

2 cups **heavy cream**

1 teaspoon **freshly grated nutmeg**

1 teaspoon **paprika**

½ teaspoon **cayenne pepper**

8 ounces **cream cheese**

½ cup shredded **provolone cheese**

There is nothing better than the heavenly aroma of bubbling, baking cheese that fills my kitchen whenever I make this dish. I normally top gratins with a crunchy layer of bread crumbs, but who needs that when you use a nice, melty cheese like provolone and bake until molten and crispy around the edges? Don't let the kale fool you; this probably won't go down as the world's healthiest food. But it is most definitely in the running for the creamiest and most comforting. Bust this out during the holidays and you'll be a hero.

1. Preheat the oven to 400°F.

2. Place a large Dutch oven over medium-high heat. Add the olive oil and heat to shimmering, then add the onion, garlic, and a pinch of salt. Cook until the vegetables are soft, stirring occasionally, about 3 minutes. Add the kale in batches, stirring occasionally to wilt it, then add the next handful, until it all fits in the pan. Cook until it has fully wilted, about 10 minutes. Drain the kale in a colander and set aside (save the pan for the next step).

3. Return to the pan to medium heat. Add the cream, nutmeg, paprika, and cayenne, whisking to combine. Cook until the liquid has reduced by half, whisking occasionally, about 5 minutes. Add the cream cheese and whisk until the cream cheese melts and the mixture is thick and creamy, about 1 minute. Season to taste with salt and black pepper.

4. Remove from the heat and stir in the kale. Top the kale with shredded provolone and bake, uncovered, until bubbling and golden brown, about 20 minutes. Serve hot or at room temperature.

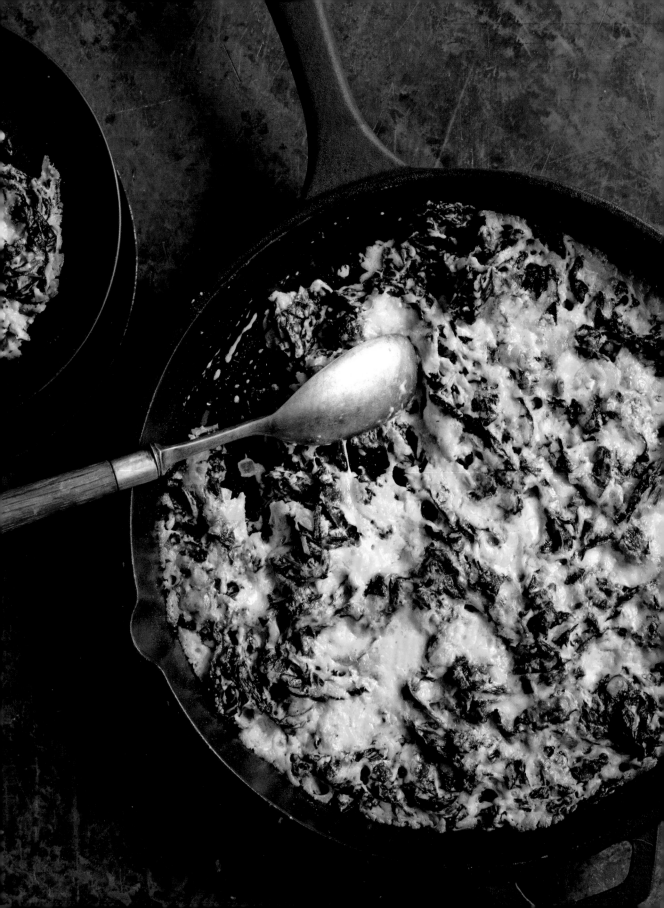

Sautéed Shrimp Summer Rolls

with Fermented Dipping Sauce

Serves 6

Summer Rolls

1 dozen medium **shrimp**, peeled and deveined

Kosher salt and freshly ground black pepper

1 tablespoon **extra-virgin olive oil**

1 **garlic clove**, grated on a rasp grater

⅛ teaspoon **dried red pepper flakes**

4 ounces **rice vermicelli noodles**

6 (8-inch) **rice paper wrappers**

½ small **red bell pepper**, thinly sliced

½ cup thinly sliced **English cucumber** (¼ of a medium cucumber)

1 cup thinly sliced **lettuce leaves**

¼ cup thinly sliced **scallions**

¼ cup finely chopped **fresh cilantro**

¼ cup finely chopped **fresh Thai basil**

¼ cup finely chopped **fresh mint**

Dipping Sauce

¼ cup **white or brown miso**

¼ cup **rice vinegar**

3 tablespoons **mirin**

2½ tablespoons **sambal oelek**

1 tablespoon **raw honey**

Liz and I can't go to a Vietnamese restaurant without ordering the summer rolls. My version is light and bright and gets a spicy kick from the sambal-based dipping sauce. You can make them a day ahead, but over time, the wrappers turn rubbery.

1. **Make the summer rolls:** Season the shrimp with salt and black pepper. In a medium bowl, whisk together the olive oil, garlic, and pepper flakes. Add the shrimp, toss to coat, and set aside.

2. Bring a medium saucepan of water to a boil. Add the noodles and cook until tender, about 3 minutes. Drain, rinse under cold water, and set aside.

3. Set a large heavy-bottomed skillet over medium-high heat. Add the shrimp and cook until well browned, about 2 minutes. Flip and brown the other side, about 2 minutes. Transfer the shrimp to a cutting board and once they are cool, halve lengthwise and set aside.

4. Fill a large bowl with warm water. Working with 1 rice wrapper at a time, dip the paper into the water until it is soft and pliable, about 30 seconds. Remove the wrapper and lay it flat on a work surface. Arrange a small portion of the rice noodles on the lower third of the wrapper. Top with a few pieces of bell pepper and cucumber, followed by a sprinkling of lettuce, scallions, cilantro, basil, and mint. Fold the bottom of the wrapper over the filling, fold the two sides in over the filling, and give the roll one turn forward. Arrange 4 slices of shrimp on top of the bundle and continue rolling forward until you have a tight roll. Repeat the process with the remaining 5 rolls. Refrigerate on a tightly wrapped plate, while you make the sauce.

5. **Make the dipping sauce:** In a medium bowl, whisk to combine the miso, rice vinegar, mirin, sambal oelek, and honey.

6. Slice the rolls diagonally and serve with dipping sauce.

Eggplant Parmesan

Serves 8

**Kosher salt and freshly ground
  black pepper**

4 medium **eggplants**, peeled
  and sliced lengthwise into
  ½-inch-thick slabs

8 tablespoons **extra-virgin olive oil**

2 cups **Pomodoro Sauce** (page 131)
  or your favorite marinara sauce,
  plus extra for serving (optional)

½ cup **freshly grated parmesan
  cheese**

½ cup thinly sliced **fresh basil leaves**

8 ounces **fresh mozzarella**, grated
  (about 2 cups)

I named my new restaurant at the Borgata
Hotel in Atlantic City after my mom, Angel. At
Angeline, the menu is an ode to Mom's home-
style cooking, which is inspired by her Greek
and Sicilian heritage. We created this dish in
her honor, and she says not only is it her favorite
item at the restaurant, she admits that it's *almost*
as good as her version. Here, I roast eggplants
instead of breading and pan-frying them for a
flour-free and healthier version of an Italian-
American classic.

1. Liberally sprinkle salt on both sides of the eggplant
slices and arrange them so they are standing up in a
colander to drain for 30 minutes. Pat the slices dry
with a kitchen towel and set aside.

2. Preheat the oven to 400°F. Line 2 sheet pans with
foil and coat the foil with 2 tablespoons of the olive oil.

3. Divide the eggplant slices between the 2 pans,
slightly overlapping them if necessary. Drizzle the
remaining 6 tablespoons olive oil over the eggplant
and season with pepper. Roast until the eggplant
slices are soft, about 12 minutes. Remove from the
oven and set aside.

4. Spread ½ cup of the pomodoro sauce evenly over
the bottom of a 9 × 13-inch baking dish. Arrange a
layer of eggplant slices across the bottom, slightly
overlapping them if necessary. Top the eggplant with
another ½ cup pomodoro sauce, followed by one-third
of the parmesan and one-half of the basil. Arrange
another layer of eggplant slices on top, followed
by ½ cup pomodoro sauce, another third of the
parmesan, all the mozzarella, and all the remaining
basil. Arrange the final layer of eggplant slices on top,
coat with the remaining ½ cup pomodoro sauce, and
evenly distribute the remaining parmesan across
the top.

▶ Recipe continues

Flour-Free Fix

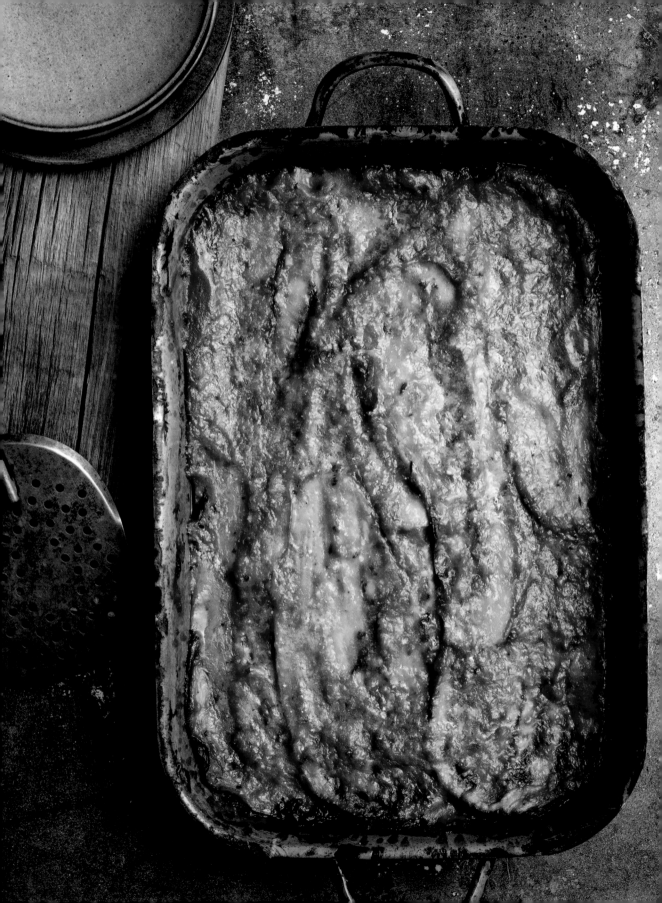

5. Cover the pan with foil and cook until the eggplant is soft throughout, about 30 minutes. Remove the foil and continue cooking until bubbling and set, about 15 minutes. Remove the pan from the oven and let rest for 15 minutes before slicing. Serve with extra pomodoro sauce, if desired.

Pomodoro Sauce

Makes 3 cups

When it's not tomato season, I live by good-quality canned San Marzano tomatoes, the next best thing. Cooking them briefly in this sauce preserves their bright and fresh flavor, which gets kissed by garlic, oregano, thyme, and sweet basil. This is my go-to quick-cook tomato sauce that goes with everything from grilled vegetables to Mom's Lasagna with Potato Noodles and Meat Sauce (page 146) to crispy Polenta with Pomodoro (page 186).

Small bunch of **fresh oregano**

Small bunch of **fresh thyme**

¼ cup **extra-virgin olive oil**

1 small **yellow onion**, finely chopped

2 **garlic cloves**, minced

¼ teaspoon **dried red pepper flakes** (optional)

Kosher salt and freshly ground black pepper

1 (28-ounce) can **whole peeled San Marzano tomatoes with juice**

½ cup torn **fresh basil leaves**

1. Bundle up the oregano and thyme in butcher's twine and set aside.

2. Place a large saucepan over medium heat. Add the olive oil and heat to shimmering, then add the onion, garlic, pepper flakes (if using), and large pinch of salt. Cook, stirring occasionally, until the vegetables soften, about 10 minutes.

3. Crush the tomatoes by hand and add them, along with their juices, to the pot. Season with a pinch of salt and a twist of black pepper and add the herb bundle. Bring the sauce to a boil, then reduce the heat to medium-low to maintain a gentle simmer and cook for 30 minutes to marry the flavors. Remove from the heat, discard the herb bundle, and lightly process in a blender until most large chunks are gone. Stir in the basil leaves. Use immediately or store refrigerated in an airtight container for up to 5 days.

Ratatouille-Baked Chicken

Serves 4

2 tablespoons **extra-virgin olive oil**

8 bone-in, skin-on **chicken thighs**

Kosher salt and freshly ground black pepper

1 small **yellow onion**, roughly chopped

5 **garlic cloves**, minced

1 large **eggplant**, peeled and cut into 1-inch cubes

1 tablespoon **tomato paste**

1 tablespoon finely chopped **fresh thyme**

2 medium **zucchini**, cut into ½-inch dice

1 **yellow bell pepper**, cut into ½-inch squares

5 **vine-ripened tomatoes**, cut into ½-inch dice

1 cup **fresh basil leaves**, finely chopped

Ratatouille is another amazing way to utilize eggplants once they start rolling into farmers' markets and gardens. This recipe elevates the classic French side dish to a main course with the addition of meaty chicken thighs. By finishing the chicken in the stew, the ratatouille gets more flavorful and the chicken stays moist and succulent: a win-win.

1. Preheat the oven to 400°F.

2. Set a large Dutch oven over medium-high heat. Add the olive oil and heat to shimmering. Pat the chicken dry with paper towels, season on all sides with salt and pepper, and set the chicken skin-side down in the pan. Cook, without moving, until nicely browned and the meat releases from the pan, about 5 minutes. Flip and continue cooking until the other side begins to brown, about 3 minutes. Remove the chicken to a plate and set aside.

3. Reduce the heat to medium and add the onion, garlic, and a pinch of salt. Cook, stirring occasionally, until the vegetables begin to soften, about 3 minutes. Add the eggplant and another pinch of salt and cook, stirring occasionally, until the eggplant begins to soften, about 5 minutes. (If the pan appears dry, add a splash of olive oil.) Add the tomato paste and thyme and cook, stirring constantly, for 1 minute. Add the zucchini, bell pepper, tomatoes, another pinch of salt, and a twist of black pepper and cook, stirring occasionally, until all of the vegetables are tender, about 10 minutes. Remove the pan from the heat.

4. Partially submerge the chicken skin-side up into the vegetables. Transfer the pot to the oven and cook, uncovered, until the thickest portion of the chicken reaches an internal temperature of 160°F, about 20 minutes. Remove from the oven and let stand for 10 minutes. Stir in the basil and serve.

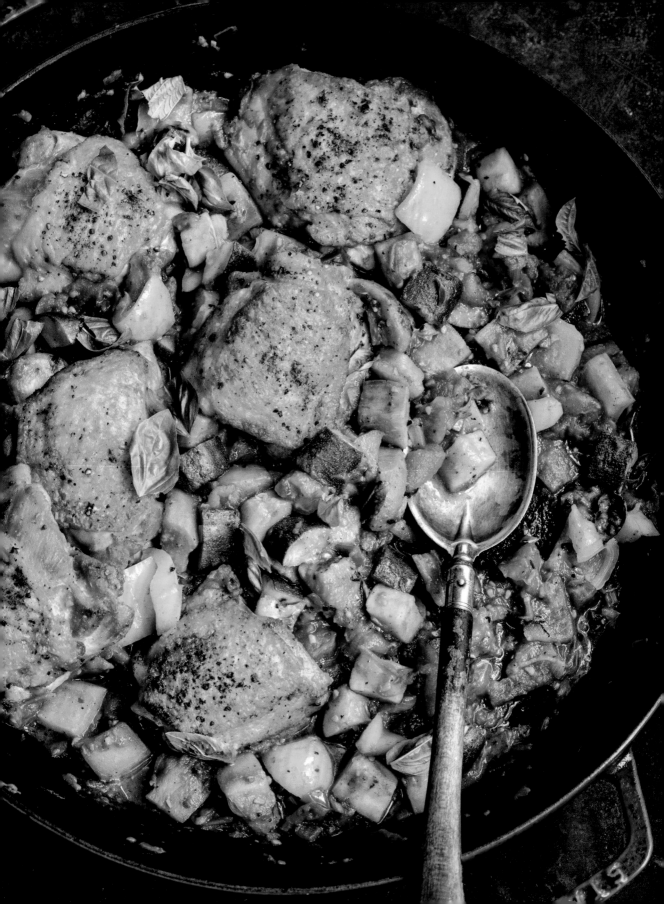

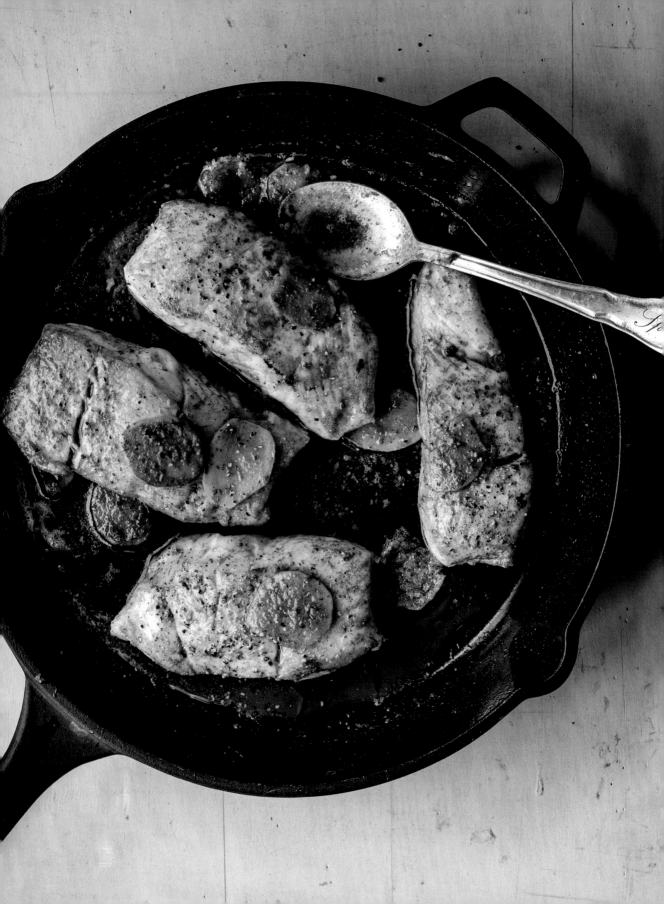

Pan-Roasted Halibut

with Turmeric Brown Butter

Serves 4

2 tablespoons **extra-virgin olive oil**

4 tablespoons **unsalted butter**

4 **halibut fillets** (6 ounces each)

Kosher salt and freshly ground black pepper

2-inch piece **fresh ginger**, peeled and thinly sliced

1 teaspoon peeled, grated **fresh turmeric** or ½ teaspoon ground turmeric

Juice of 1 lemon

As I have mentioned throughout this book, turmeric is a remarkable anti-inflammatory ingredient that helps me cope with my arthritis. Therefore, I try to come up with new and different ways to incorporate it into recipes. This one works great because it blends in seamlessly with the brown butter. I use a technique called pan-basting here—you've likely seen chefs on TV do it. It's a great way to cook fish because it improves moisture, flavor, and texture with little risk of overcooking. The halibut would go great with Spring Pea Hummus (page 220), and if you can't find halibut or are looking for a less expensive fish, try wild striped bass or cod.

1. Set a large heavy-bottomed skillet over medium heat. Add the olive oil and butter. Using paper towels, pat the halibut fillets dry. Season the fish on all sides with salt and add to the pan, making sure to leave space between the pieces. Cook, without moving, until nicely browned and the fish releases from the pan, about 3 minutes. Flip and continue cooking for 3 minutes. Move the fish to one side of the pan.

2. To the open space in the pan, add the ginger and turmeric. Carefully tilt the pan so that the butter sauce pools to the side with the ginger. With a spoon, baste the fish with the sauce until the butter has browned and begins to froth, about 2 minutes. Add the lemon juice and ½ teaspoon black pepper to the pan and continue basting the fish until the flesh turns opaque and begins to flake, about 2 minutes.

3. Remove the fish to a platter, discard the ginger, drizzle with any remaining sauce, and serve.

Baked Bass Shakshuka-Style

Serves 4

3 tablespoons **extra-virgin olive oil**

1 small **yellow onion**, halved and thinly sliced

1 **red bell pepper**, thinly sliced

3 **garlic cloves**, thinly sliced

1 **jalapeño**, thinly sliced into rings

Kosher salt and freshly ground black pepper

1 teaspoon **ground cumin**

1 teaspoon **paprika**

⅛ teaspoon **cayenne pepper**

1 (28-ounce) can **crushed San Marzano tomatoes**

1 to 2 teaspoons **sherry vinegar**, to taste

4 **striped bass fillets** (6 ounces each)

The Middle Eastern (some say North African) dish shakshuka is all the rage these days, but I've been making (and loving) it for years. It's a simple one-skillet dish where eggs are poached in a spicy tomato sauce or flavorful braised greens like Baked Eggs with Mushrooms, Collards, and Onions (page 173) in the Meat-Free Fix chapter. This version swaps the eggs for plump fillets of striped bass, transforming a popular brunch dish into a delicious dinner. This technique is great for cooking delicate fish because it keeps the fish moist while imparting flavor.

1. Preheat the oven to 400°F.

2. Set a large Dutch oven over medium heat. Add the olive oil and heat to shimmering, then add the onion, bell pepper, garlic, jalapeño, and a pinch of salt. Cook, stirring occasionally, until the vegetables are tender and beginning to brown, about 3 minutes. Add the cumin, paprika, and cayenne and cook, stirring constantly, for 1 minute. Add the tomatoes along with their juices, season with another pinch of salt and a twist of black pepper, and bring to a boil. Reduce the heat to medium-low to maintain a gentle simmer, partially cover, and cook until the vegetables soften and the liquid has mostly reduced, about 30 minutes.

3. Remove from the heat and stir in the vinegar. Season the fish on all sides with salt and black pepper and partially submerge in the sauce, leaving space between the pieces. Transfer the pot to the oven and cook, uncovered, until the flesh of the fish turns opaque and begins to flake, about 15 minutes.

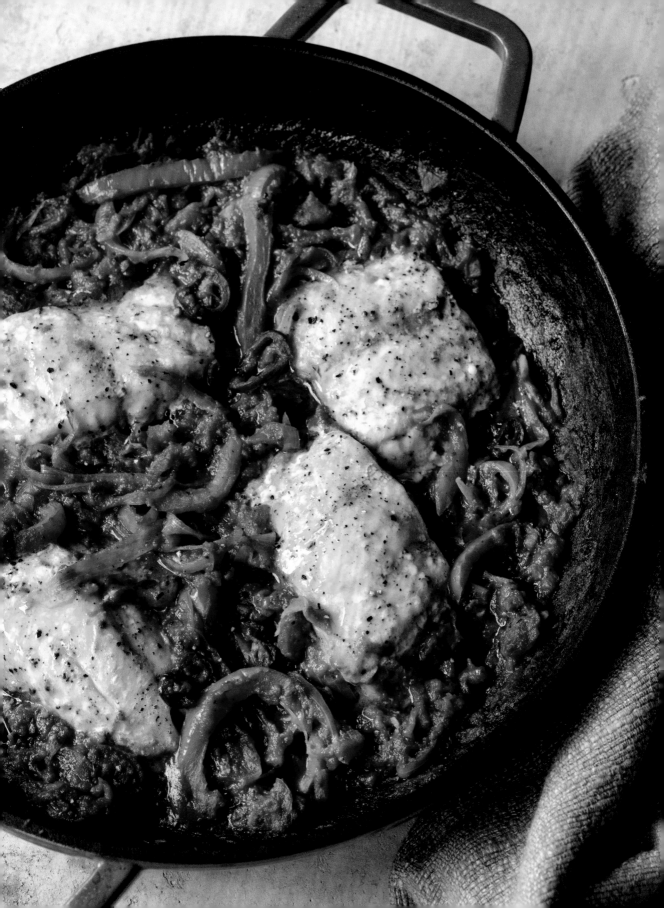

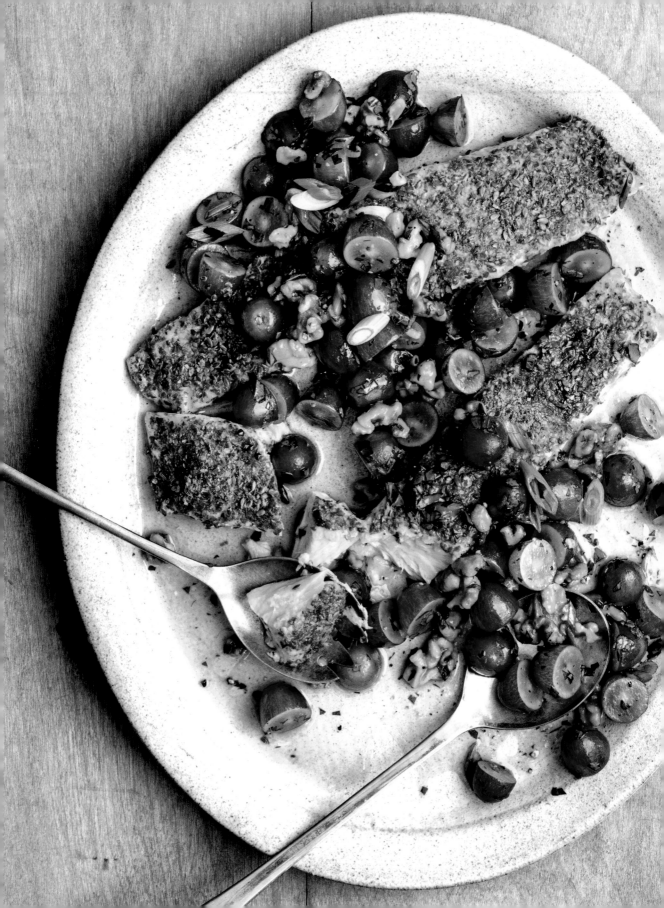

Flaxseed-Crusted Salmon

with a Grape and Walnut Salsa

Serves 4

1 cup **walnut halves**

4 **skin-on salmon fillets** (6 ounces each), pin bones removed

2 tablespoons **Dijon mustard**

Kosher salt and freshly ground black pepper

2 tablespoons **ground flaxseed**

8 tablespoons **extra-virgin olive oil**

2 tablespoons **red wine vinegar**

1 tablespoon **raw honey**

3 cups **seedless red grapes**, halved

½ cup chopped **fresh flat-leaf parsley**

2 **scallions**, thinly sliced

I'm not sure you could design a recipe healthier than this dish—this one truly has it all, from good fats to protein, and fiber to antioxidants. Equally important is the fact that it's effortless to make and tastes amazing. Roasting fish on a sheet pan in a hot oven simplifies the cooking process, while the grape and walnut salsa keeps things light, bright, fresh, and crunchy and flaxseeds take the place of bread crumbs. Did I mention that it's just as great at room temperature or even cold from the fridge as it is warm? I remember eating this on set and being amazed at how well it held up from the day before!

1. Preheat the oven to 350°F.

2. Place the walnuts on a sheet pan and cook until lightly toasted, about 8 minutes. Transfer the walnuts to a cutting board and when cool enough to handle, roughly chop and set aside.

3. Increase the oven temperature to 400°F. Line a sheet pan with foil.

4. Using paper towels, pat the fish fillets dry. Evenly coat each salmon fillet with ½ tablespoon of the mustard. Season the fillets on all sides with salt and pepper and then sprinkle ½ tablespoon of the flaxseed on top of each piece of fish, gently pressing them into the flesh. Place the fish on the lined sheet pan and drizzle each fillet with 1 tablespoon of the olive oil. Transfer to the oven and bake until the fish reaches an internal temperature of 125°F, about 10 minutes.

5. Meanwhile, in a medium bowl, whisk together the remaining 4 tablespoons olive oil, the vinegar, and honey. Season with a pinch of salt and a twist of black pepper. Add the walnuts, grapes, parsley, and scallions and toss together.

6. When the fish is done, remove it from the oven, top each piece with a generous amount of salsa, and serve.

Chicken Meatball Bourguignon

Serves 6

Meatballs

3 tablespoons **extra-virgin olive oil**

1 small **yellow onion**, finely chopped

2 **garlic cloves**, minced

Kosher salt and freshly ground black pepper

1 pound **ground chicken**

½ cup **gluten-free bread crumbs**

½ cup **flat-leaf parsley leaves**, finely chopped

1 teaspoon **dried oregano**

1 large **egg**, lightly beaten

1 tablespoon **Worcestershire sauce**

⅓ cup **freshly grated parmesan cheese**

This recipe is a twist on the classic beef Bourguignon from Burgundy, France. I swap the beef with flavorful chicken meatballs, which adds a little work but is oh-so worth it. Make this dish for a wintertime dinner party and your friends will never forget it. You should always cook with wine that is good enough to drink, and this is no exception. Look for a good-quality pinot noir and grab an extra bottle or two to drink. Serve this dish over some simple mashed potatoes. The meatballs can be made a day ahead and refrigerated overnight.

1. **Make the meatballs:** Set a medium heavy-bottomed skillet over medium-high heat. Add 1 tablespoon of the olive oil and heat to shimmering, then add the onion, garlic, and a pinch of salt. Cook, stirring occasionally, until the vegetables soften, about 5 minutes. Remove from the heat to cool slightly.

2. In a large bowl, combine the chicken, bread crumbs, parsley, oregano, egg, Worcestershire, and parmesan and stir to combine. Add the cooked onion mixture, season with a pinch of salt and a twist of pepper, and mix. Form the mixture into 12 equal meatballs about the size of a golf ball and chill until needed. (This can be done a day ahead.)

3. Set a large Dutch oven over medium-high heat. Add the remaining 2 tablespoons olive oil. When hot add the meatballs and cook, turning occasionally, until browned on all sides, about 8 minutes. Remove from the pan and set aside.

Stew

4 strips **thick-sliced bacon**

2 medium **yellow onions**, finely chopped

1 cup (½-inch pieces) **carrot**

1 cup (½-inch pieces) **celery**

2 **garlic cloves**, minced

1 tablespoon **tomato paste**

1 tablespoon **thyme leaves**

3 cups **Beef Bone Broth** (page 237)

2 cups **dry red wine**

5 tablespoons **unsalted butter**, at room temperature

2 cups quartered **cremini mushrooms**

1 cup peeled and quartered **cipollini onions**

3 tablespoons **rice flour**

½ cup **flat-leaf parsley leaves**, roughly chopped

4. **Make the stew:** Discard any fat from the pan and return it to the heat. Add the bacon and cook, stirring occasionally, until crisp, about 3 minutes. Add the onions, carrot, celery, and garlic and cook, stirring occasionally, until the vegetables soften, about 4 minutes. Add the tomato paste and thyme and cook, stirring occasionally, for 1 minute. Add the bone broth and wine and bring to a gentle boil. Reduce the heat to a simmer, add the meatballs, and cook, stirring occasionally, until the meatballs are fully cooked, about 30 minutes.

5. Meanwhile, place a large heavy-bottomed skillet over high heat. Add 2 tablespoons of the butter and once melted, arrange the mushrooms and cipollini onions so they are in a single layer on the bottom of the pan. Cook, stirring minimally, until deep golden brown, about 8 minutes. Season with a pinch of salt and a twist of black pepper and add the mushroom mixture to the meatballs.

6. In a medium bowl, combine the remaining 3 tablespoons of softened butter with the rice flour to form a paste. Whisk the paste into the stew a little bit at a time until it's all combined. Continue cooking the stew, stirring occasionally, until thickened and glossy, about 5 minutes. Remove from the heat and stir in the parsley. Taste and add salt and pepper if needed.

Yogurt-Roasted Chicken

Serves 4

1 cup **whole-milk Greek yogurt**

4 tablespoons **extra-virgin olive oil**

2 **garlic cloves**, minced

2 tablespoons grated **fresh ginger**

½ teaspoon **ground cinnamon**

½ teaspoon **cayenne pepper**

2 tablespoons chopped **fresh cilantro**

Grated zest and juice of 1 orange

1 large **chicken** (4 to 6 pounds), preferably organic

Kosher salt and freshly ground black pepper

Yogurt makes an ideal marinade for chicken. Its natural acidity tenderizes the meat, infuses it with flavorful spices and aromatics, and produces a golden brown, Instagram-worthy skin that will impress your guests (and social media followers). If you have the time to marinate the bird overnight, the results will be ten times better! If you somehow don't eat the whole thing at dinnertime, you probably will by lunch the next day.

1. In a medium bowl, whisk together the yogurt, 2 tablespoons of the olive oil, the garlic, ginger, cinnamon, cayenne, cilantro, orange zest, and orange juice. Pat the chicken dry with paper towels and then add it to the bowl with the marinade. Liberally coat the inside and outside with the marinade, and refrigerate the chicken in the bowl, uncovered, for at least 2 hours, but preferably overnight.

2. Remove the chicken from the refrigerator and allow it to come to room temperature, about 30 minutes.

3. Preheat the oven to 375°F. Set a roasting rack on a rimmed sheet pan and set aside.

4. Remove the chicken from the marinade, wiping off most but not all of the yogurt, and place it on the rack. Drizzle the chicken with the remaining 2 tablespoons olive oil, season with a few pinches of salt and twists of black pepper, and roast, uncovered, for 1 hour. Baste the chicken with any pan juices and continue roasting until the thickest portion of the thigh reaches an internal temperature of 160°F, about 20 minutes.

5. Transfer the chicken to a cutting board and let it rest for 15 minutes before carving and serving.

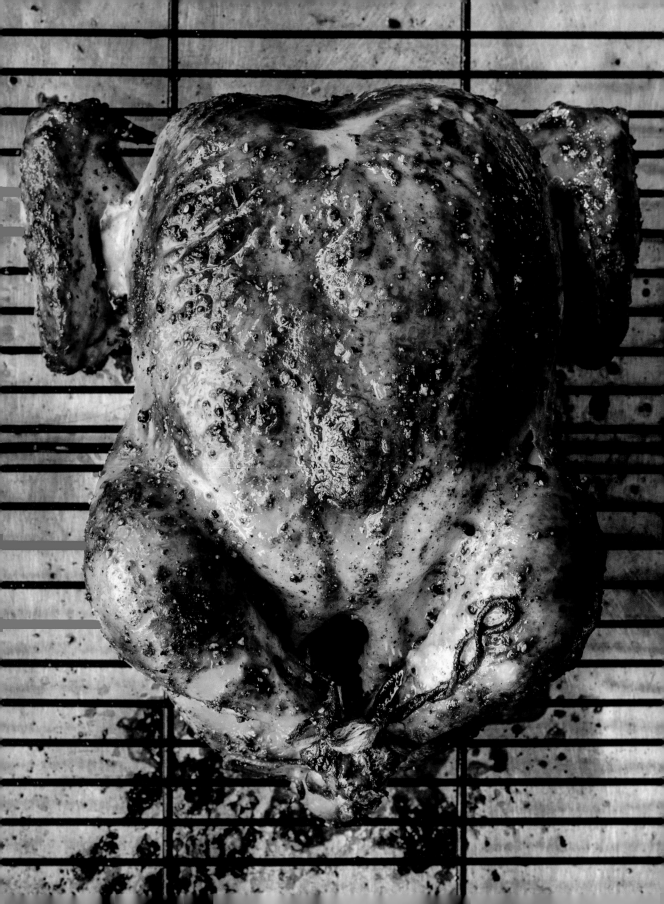

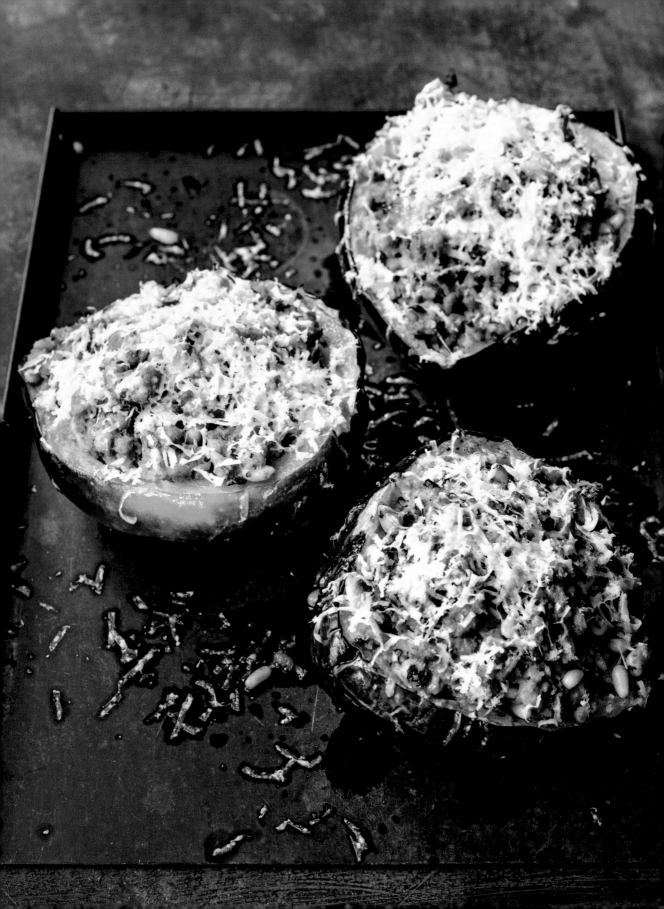

Baked Acorn Squash

Stuffed with Ground Turkey and Pine Nuts

Serves 6

½ cup **pine nuts**

3 **acorn squash**, halved and seeded

Extra-virgin olive oil

Kosher salt and freshly ground black pepper

1½ pounds **ground turkey**

1 small **red onion**, finely chopped

2 **garlic cloves**, minced

½ teaspoon **ground cinnamon**

½ cup chopped **fresh flat-leaf parsley**

1 cup **freshly grated Pecorino-Romano cheese**

Nothing says autumn like heavenly roasted acorn squash. This mild-tasting cold-weather squash is perfect for stuffing because of its bowl-like shape, which is even fluted for an attractive presentation. The nutty-sweet flesh goes great with savory fillings like this one, and that golden hue means that it's loaded with beta-carotene.

1. Preheat the oven to 350°F.

2. Place the pine nuts on a sheet pan and cook until lightly toasted, about 6 minutes. Transfer the pine nuts to a plate.

3. Increase the oven temperature to 400°F. Line the sheet pan with foil.

4. Place the squash on the foil-lined pan and coat the exposed flesh with olive oil, season with a pinch of salt and a twist of black pepper, and turn the squash cut-side down. Cook until the squash is easily pierced with a knife, about 45 minutes. Remove from the oven, flip the squash so it's cut-side up, scoop about one-third of the flesh from each squash, and set aside.

5. Set a large heavy-bottomed skillet over high heat. Add a drizzle of olive oil and heat to shimmering, then add the turkey and cook, stirring with a wooden spoon to break up the meat, until lightly browned, about 2 minutes. Add the onion and garlic, season with a pinch of salt and a twist of black pepper, and continue cooking until the vegetables soften, about 2 minutes. Add the toasted pine nuts and cinnamon and stir to combine. Remove from the heat, add the scooped-out and reserved squash, and stir in the parsley and half of the pecorino.

6. Divide the turkey mixture evenly among the squash, mounding it into the cavities. Divide the remaining cheese over the tops and cook until warmed through, about 5 minutes. Remove from the oven, drizzle with olive oil, and serve.

Flour-Free Fix

145

Mom's Lasagna

with Potato Noodles and Meat Sauce

Serves 8

1 tablespoon **extra-virgin olive oil**

1 pound **80% lean ground beef**

Kosher salt and freshly ground black pepper

Pomodoro Sauce (page 131) or 3½ cups of your favorite store-bought marinara

2 large **eggs**

2 pounds **whole-milk ricotta cheese**

¼ cup finely chopped **fresh flat-leaf parsley**

¼ cup finely chopped **fresh oregano**

¼ cup finely chopped **fresh basil**

3 pounds **Yukon Gold potatoes**, peeled and cut crosswise into ⅛-inch-thick slices

8 ounces **fresh mozzarella**, grated (about 2 cups)

¼ cup **freshly grated parmesan cheese**

My deathbed meal would probably be my mom's lasagna—it's that good. This is a flour-free version that I came up with by substituting thinly sliced potatoes for the pasta noodles. It might anger pasta purists, but I think it tastes amazing (and if you want to try Mom's original version, the recipe can easily be found online). If you don't have a vegetable slicer or a mandoline, I suggest that you consider investing in one. For about $25, you can breeze your way to paper-thin slices for recipes like this one and many others, including Shaved Beet Salad (page 105), Cauliflower Salad with Apples, Pistachios, and Goji Berries (page 165), or the shaved Brussels sprouts in the Brussels Sprouts, Apple, and Brown Rice Salad (page 73).

1. Set a large heavy-bottomed skillet over medium-high heat. Add the olive oil and heat to shimmering, then add the ground beef. Cook until well browned, stirring occasionally to break up the meat, about 5 minutes. Drain the fat from the pan. Season the meat with a pinch of salt and a twist of black pepper, stir in the pomodoro sauce, and bring to a simmer. Taste and add salt and pepper if needed. Remove from the heat and set aside.

2. Preheat the oven to 375°F. Line a sheet pan with foil.

3. In a large bowl, beat the eggs and then whisk in the ricotta, parsley, oregano, and basil and season with a pinch of salt and a twist of black pepper. Set aside.

4. Spread 1 cup of the meat sauce evenly over the bottom of a 9 × 13-inch baking dish. Season all of the potato slices with salt and pepper. Arrange a layer of potatoes across the bottom, slightly overlapping them. Top the potatoes with another 1 cup of the meat sauce, followed by one-third of the ricotta

▶ Recipe continues

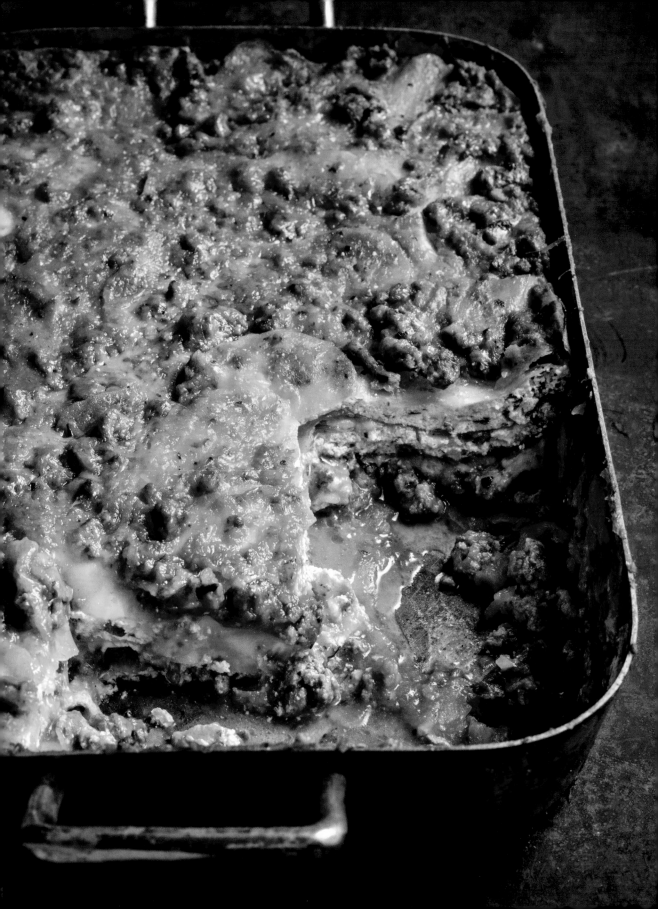

cheese mixture, and then one-half of the mozzarella. Arrange another layer of overlapping potato slices on top, pressing them down gently. Top the potatoes with another 1 cup of the meat sauce, another one-third of the ricotta cheese mixture, and all the remaining mozzarella. Arrange another layer of overlapping potato slices, pressing them down gently. Top with the remaining ricotta cheese mixture and a final layer of overlapping potato slices. Top with the rest of the meat sauce and evenly distribute the parmesan across the top.

5. Coat a piece of foil with cooking spray and set it, sprayed-side down, over the lasagna, crimping down the edges. Place the baking dish on the lined sheet pan and bake until the potatoes are easily pierced with a knife, about 1½ hours. Uncover the lasagna and continue cooking until the top of the lasagna is slightly browned, about 15 minutes. Remove from the oven and let rest for 10 minutes before slicing and serving.

Cast-Iron Strip Steaks

with Red Wine and Roasted Garlic Butter Sauce

Serves 4

1 head **garlic**, loose papery skins removed

1 tablespoon **extra-virgin olive oil**, plus more for cooking

4 **strip steaks** (12 ounces each)

Kosher salt and freshly ground black pepper

½ cup **dry red wine**

2 tablespoons **fresh rosemary** leaves, finely chopped

4 tablespoons **unsalted butter**, cubed and chilled

1 teaspoon **fresh lemon juice**

Ask my neighbors—I'm the crazy guy who grills outdoors all winter long. But even I have my limits. So when I want to cook a deeply charred and juicy steak without having to lace up my winter boots, this is my favorite method. Open the windows, preheat the pan (cast-iron works best), turn on the vent fan, liberally season the meat, and bust out the instant-read thermometer (please tell me that you own an instant-read thermometer). I'm getting hungry just thinking about it! For a great chophouse meal, serve this with Skillet Kale Gratin (page 126).

1. Preheat the oven to 400°F.

2. Slice the top ¼ inch off the garlic head to expose some of the cloves. Place the garlic head cut-side up in a large piece of foil, drizzle with the 1 tablespoon olive oil, and form a loose packet by gathering the foil up around the garlic. Place directly on the oven rack and cook until the garlic is fragrant, golden brown, and soft, about 45 minutes. Remove the packet from the oven, carefully open the foil, and set aside to cool.

3. Meanwhile, remove the steaks from the refrigerator, discard any packaging, and allow them to come to room temperature, about 20 minutes.

4. Set a large heavy-bottomed skillet over medium heat. Add a drizzle of olive oil to the pan and swirl to coat. Pat the steaks dry with paper towels and then liberally season them on both sides with salt and pepper and add them to the pan, making sure to leave some space between them. Cook, without moving, until nicely browned and the steaks release from the pan, about 6 minutes. Flip and continue cooking until the meat reaches an internal temperature of 130°F for medium-rare, about 5 minutes. Remove the steaks to a cutting board and loosely tent with foil.

▶ Recipe continues

Flour-Free Fix

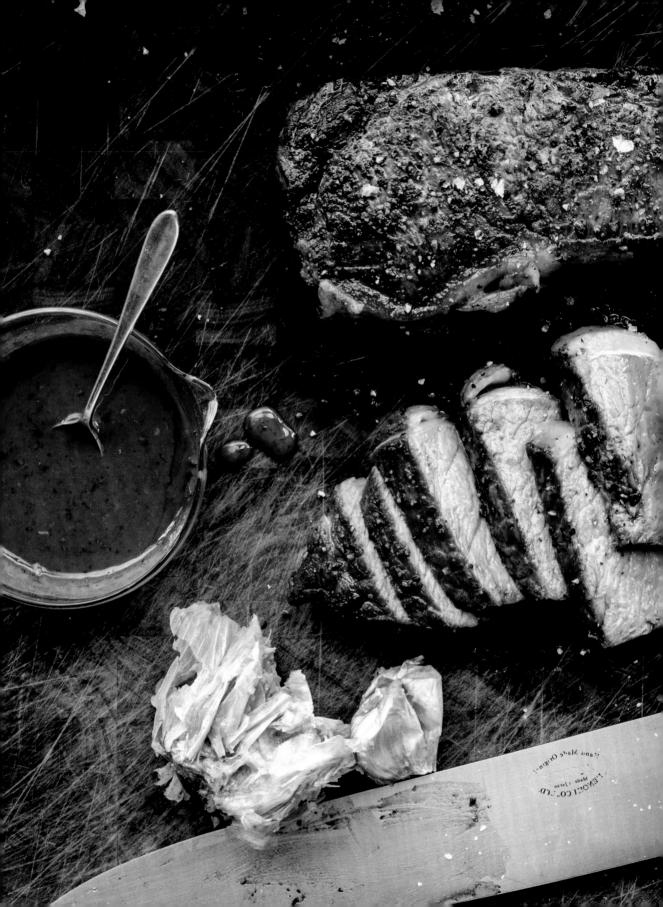

5. Discard any remaining fat from the pan and return it to medium heat. Add the wine and deglaze the pan, scraping with a wooden spoon to get up the browned bits on the bottom of the pan. Squeeze the roasted garlic directly from the head into the pan, followed by the rosemary. Cook, stirring occasionally, until the liquid is reduced by half and the garlic has broken down into the sauce, about 2 minutes.

6. Remove the pan from the heat and whisk in the butter. Stir in the lemon juice and season with a pinch of salt and a twist of black pepper. Slice the steaks against the grain and serve drizzled with the sauce.

Curried Lentils

with Lamb and Sweet Potatoes

Serves 6

2 pounds **lamb stew or shoulder meat**, cut into 1-inch cubes

½ teaspoon **ground cinnamon**

½ teaspoon **ground cumin**

Kosher salt and freshly ground black pepper

3 tablespoons **extra-virgin olive oil**

1 medium **red onion**, diced

2 **garlic cloves**, minced

1 tablespoon grated **fresh ginger**

4 cups **Beef Bone Broth** (page 237)

2 cups **brown lentils**, rinsed

2 **sweet potatoes**, peeled and cut into 1-inch cubes

1 cup **Turmeric Milk** (page 245)

Grated zest and juice of 1 orange

1 cup chopped **fresh cilantro**

Thinly sliced **scallions**, for serving (optional)

There is just so much deliciousness going on in this recipe. The combination of lamb, curry, and sweet potatoes is magical, and the lentils absorb and retain all those amazing flavors. If you don't like or have easy access to lamb stew meat, feel free to swap it out for beef chuck, pork shoulder, or turkey thighs. Serve this as a savory stew with Kyle's Coconut Rice (page 106) and you'll be in heaven.

1. In a large bowl, toss together the lamb, cinnamon, cumin, a pinch of salt, and a twist of black pepper.

2. Set a large Dutch oven over medium-high heat. Add the olive oil and heat to shimmering, then add the lamb in a single layer. Cook, stirring occasionally, until nicely browned on all sides, about 10 minutes. Add the onion, garlic, ginger, and a pinch of salt and continue cooking until the vegetables begin to soften, about 3 minutes. Add the bone broth, 4 cups water, and the lentils. Bring to a boil, reduce the heat to maintain a gentle simmer, and cook, partially covered and stirring occasionally, until the lentils are tender, about 45 minutes.

3. Add the sweet potatoes and turmeric milk and continue cooking, partially covered and stirring occasionally, until the lamb, lentils, and sweet potatoes are completely tender, about 1 hour more.

4. Remove from the heat and stir in the orange zest and orange juice. Taste, add salt and pepper if needed, and finish with cilantro and scallions (if using).

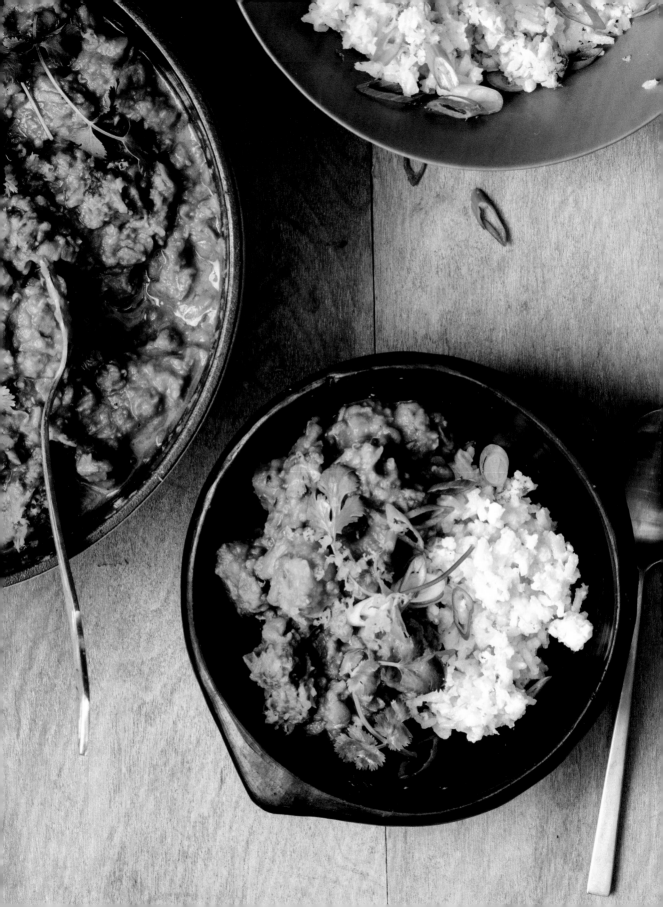

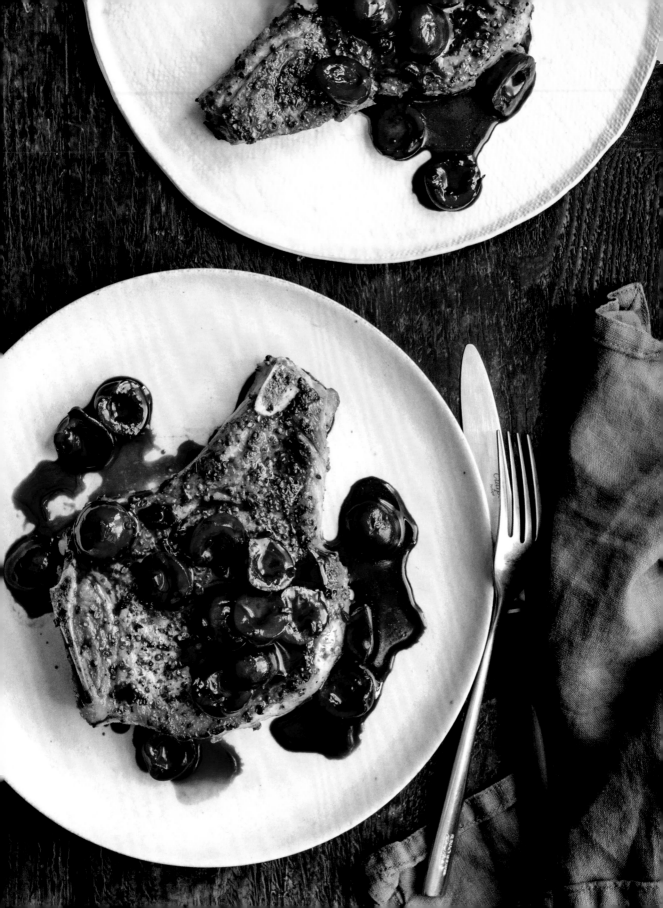

Sour Cherry Glazed Pork Chops

Serves 4

4 **bone-in pork rib chops**
(10 ounces each)

**Kosher salt and freshly ground
black pepper**

2 tablespoons **crushed coriander
seeds** (see note)

2 tablespoons **extra-virgin olive oil**

2 cups pitted fresh or frozen **tart
cherries**

1 **shallot**, finely chopped

2-inch piece **fresh ginger**, peeled
and sliced crosswise into thirds

1 cup **dry red wine**

1 **whole star anise**

1 **fresh bay leaf**

1 cup **Beef Bone Broth** (page 237)

1 tablespoon **red wine vinegar**

1 tablespoon **raw honey**

1 tablespoon **unsalted butter**

Note To crush coriander seeds, put the whole seeds in a zip-top bag and place a heavy-bottomed skillet or pot on top. Press down to gently crush the seeds.

To me, there are few flavor combinations better than pork and fruit. The earthy-sweet meat has long been paired with apples, which provide a mellow tartness that slices through the richness. I push that concept even further by using sour cherries, an underutilized ingredient if ever there was one. With the addition of honey, this sauce takes on a little sweet-and-sour action that makes the chops sing. As an added bonus, sour cherries are high in antioxidants. You can find them in-season spring through summer depending on where you live, but frozen cherries work almost as well.

1. Pat the pork dry with paper towels, season both sides with salt and pepper, and evenly coat both sides with coriander.

2. Set a large heavy-bottomed skillet over medium-high heat. Add the olive oil and heat to shimmering, then add the pork chops, making sure to leave space between the pieces. Cook, without moving, until nicely browned and the meat releases from the pan, about 4 minutes. Flip and continue cooking until the second side is nicely charred, about 4 minutes. Remove the chops to a platter and loosely tent with foil.

3. Discard all but 2 tablespoons of fat from the skillet and return it to medium heat. Add the cherries, shallot, and ginger and cook, stirring occasionally, for 1 minute. Add the wine, star anise, and bay leaf and cook until half of the liquid has evaporated, about 5 minutes. Add the bone broth and vinegar and cook until half of the liquid has evaporated, about 5 minutes. Season with a pinch of salt and a twist of black pepper.

4. Remove the pan from the heat, discard the star anise, bay leaf, and large pieces of ginger and stir in the honey and butter. Top the pork chops with the cherry sauce and serve.

Meat-Free Free Fix

Coming from the guy who wrote the cookbook called *Carnivore,* **operates two Mabel's BBQ restaurants where one of the most popular items is called "Giant Beef Ribs," and runs a small chain of B Spot hamburger joints, it's safe to assume that I love meat!** I'm not sure how (or if) I would survive if forced to permanently give up meat. Luckily, red meats like beef, pork, and lamb do not adversely affect me the way that dairy, sugar, and processed flours do.

Just because I love and have few problems with red (and white) meat doesn't mean that I eat meat at every meal. Far from it, in fact. My wife, Lizzie, has been meat-free for ages and never felt great after eating red meat; this has forced me to adjust the way I live, eat, and cook. Over the years, my appreciation for vegan and vegetarian dishes has continued to grow, mainly because I'm doing most of the cooking! I can assure you that the recipes in this chapter won't leave you wishing for bacon, spare ribs, a lamb chop, skirt steak, or . . . well, you get the idea.

Believe me, I still enjoy red meat on a consistent basis, but I tend to cook smaller portions and balance it out with plenty of fruits, vegetables, grains, beans, and eggs. I know I sound like a broken record, but moderation really is the key to being healthy and feeling great. Because I'm often cooking for and with a vegetarian, these recipes are also nutritionally balanced with plenty of protein and good carbohydrates. I think people would be surprised by how much protein there is in foods like spinach, beans, quinoa, and flax.

Because these recipes don't have the benefits of animal fat to provide flavor, it's important not to skimp on aromatics like herbs, spices, and seasonings. Fresh herbs, good-quality (and recently purchased) spices, homemade vegetable stock, last-minute additions of citrus, and punchy vinaigrettes transform what are often (in my opinion) bland and boring vegetarian dishes into satisfying and even exciting ones. There's good reason why plant-based and plant-forward restaurants are all the rage right now in big cities across the country.

Spinach and Phyllo Pies

Serves 8

4 tablespoons **extra-virgin olive oil**

2 pounds **spinach leaves**

Kosher salt and freshly ground black pepper

½ cup **pine nuts**

1 small **yellow onion**, finely chopped

2 **garlic cloves**, minced

½ teaspoon **dried red pepper flakes**

½ cup **fresh dill**, finely chopped

½ cup crumbled **feta cheese**

Grated zest of 1 lemon

4 sheets frozen **phyllo dough**, thawed

6 tablespoons **unsalted butter**, melted

My mom is the queen when it comes to making spanakopita triangles, one of my all-time favorite foods while growing up. The shatteringly crisp phyllo gives way to a soft, lemony spinach center dotted with salty feta. For holidays and get-togethers, she'd crank out dozens and dozens at our kitchen island before my sister and I could produce even a few. They're fun to form when you get the hang of it: no different from the paper footballs we used to make (and flick) in class. You can store the well-wrapped pies in the freezer for up to 4 months before baking.

1. Set a large skillet over medium-high heat. Add 1 tablespoon of the olive oil and heat to shimmering, then add the spinach leaves and a pinch of salt. Cook, stirring occasionally, until completely wilted, about 2 minutes. Drain the spinach in a fine-mesh sieve, lightly pushing it with the back of a spoon to expel excess liquid. Set aside.

2. Preheat the oven to 350°F.

3. Spread the pine nuts on a sheet pan and cook until lightly toasted, about 8 minutes. Set aside. Increase the oven temperature to 375°F.

4. Set a large heavy-bottomed skillet over medium heat. Add the remaining 3 tablespoons olive oil and heat to shimmering, then add the onion, garlic, and a pinch of salt. Cook, stirring occasionally, until the onion begins to soften, about 2 minutes. Remove from the heat and stir in the pine nuts, pepper flakes, and dill. Let cool completely, about 10 minutes.

5. In a large bowl, combine the spinach, feta, lemon zest, and cooled pine nut mixture. Season with a pinch of salt and a twist of black pepper and toss to combine.

6. Line a sheet pan with parchment paper. On a work surface, cut the 4 sheets of phyllo in half lengthwise so you have 8 strips. Keep them covered with a slightly

damp kitchen towel while assembling the individual pies. Working with one strip at a time, brush the phyllo with melted butter, place 1 tablespoon of the filling on the end closest to you, and fold over the dough to form a small triangle and enclose the filling. Continue folding the packet over itself as if folding up a flag until you reach the end of the phyllo. Place seam-side down on the lined sheet pan and brush with melted butter. Repeat with the remaining 7 strips of phyllo.

7.   Bake until the phyllo is crisp and golden brown, about 10 minutes. Remove from the oven and let stand for 5 minutes before serving.

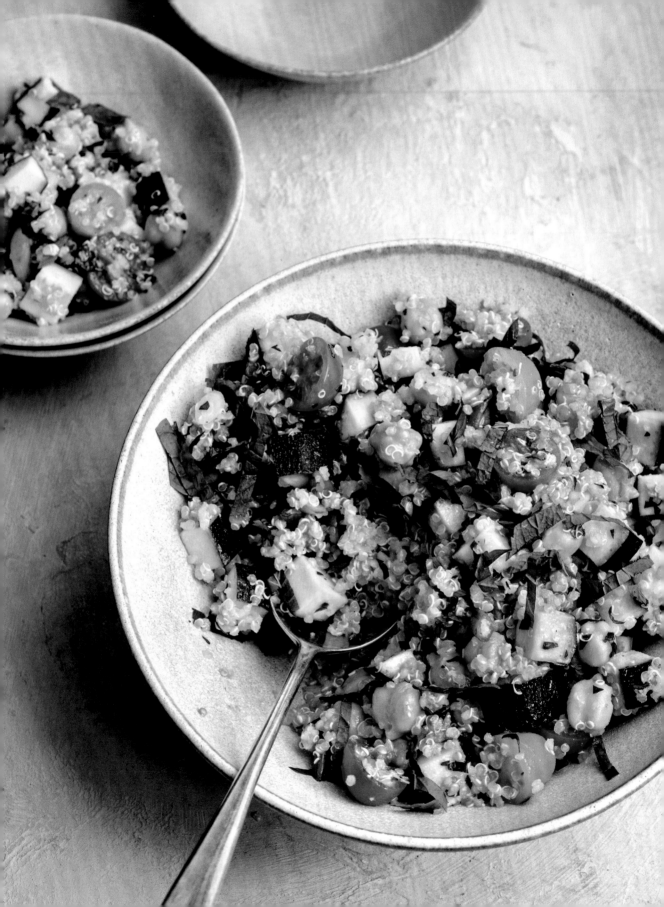

Zucchini, Chickpea, and Quinoa Salad

Serves 6

1 cup **quinoa**, rinsed

Kosher salt and freshly ground black pepper

½ cup **extra-virgin olive oil**

⅓ cup **fresh lemon juice** (about 2 lemons)

1 teaspoon **Dijon mustard**

2 medium **zucchini**, cut into ¼-inch dice

1 pint **grape tomatoes**, halved

1 (15-ounce) can **chickpeas**, drained and rinsed

¼ cup **fresh mint leaves**, finely chopped

¼ cup **fresh flat-leaf parsley**, finely chopped

¼ cup **fresh basil leaves**, thinly sliced

1 bunch **scallions**, thinly sliced

Once you get the hang of cooking quinoa, you'll go out of your way to find new uses for it. It's light, fluffy, and pleasantly nutty, which makes it a perfect base for hearty salads like this one. Plus, you can make a big batch early in the week and keep it in the fridge—it keeps its texture and moistness for nearly a week. This gluten-free grain (actually a seed) is packed with vitamins and minerals, but also flavonoids like quercetin and kaempferol, which are powerful antioxidants. Add in chickpeas, a reliable source of protein and fiber, and you've got a truly super food.

1. In a medium saucepan, combine 1¾ cups water, the quinoa, and a pinch of salt. Bring to a boil over high heat, then reduce the heat to medium-low to maintain a gentle simmer. Cook, partially covered, until the quinoa pops open and becomes tender, about 15 minutes. Remove from the heat and set aside, uncovered.

2. In a large bowl, whisk to combine the olive oil, lemon juice, and mustard. Season with a pinch of salt and a twist of black pepper. Add the cooked quinoa, zucchini, tomatoes, chickpeas, mint, parsley, basil, and scallions and toss together. Taste and add salt and pepper if needed.

Spring Pea Tabbouleh

Serves 4

¼ cup **bulgur wheat**

½ cup **boiling water**

Kosher salt and freshly ground black pepper

2 cups fresh or frozen **peas**

½ cup **extra-virgin olive oil**

Grated zest and juice of 3 lemons

3 cups finely chopped **flat-leaf parsley**

½ cup finely chopped **mint**

¼ cup finely sliced **scallions**

In the spring, the peas that I grow in my garden usually get eaten straight out of the pod—while I'm still in the garden! When I have the willpower to save a few, this is one of my favorite nutritious ways to use them. Classic tabbouleh made with bulgur wheat is terrific as is, but the addition of impeccably sweet English peas just takes it to another level—a ton of lemon juice and mint add to the appeal as well.

1. In a small heatproof bowl, combine the bulgur and boiling water. Cover and let sit until the bulgur is softened, 20 to 30 minutes. Drain well.

2. Meanwhile, prepare an ice bath by filling a medium bowl with ice and water. Fill a medium saucepan with water, add 1 tablespoon salt, and bring to a boil over high heat. Add the peas and cook until just tender, about 1 minute. Drain the peas in a colander and immediately plunge them into the ice bath to cool. Once cooled, drain again and briefly allow to dry on a kitchen towel.

3. In a medium bowl, whisk together the olive oil, lemon zest, and lemon juice. Add the bulgur, peas, parsley, mint, and scallions and toss together. Season to taste with salt and pepper. Can be made a few hours in advance and stored in the fridge.

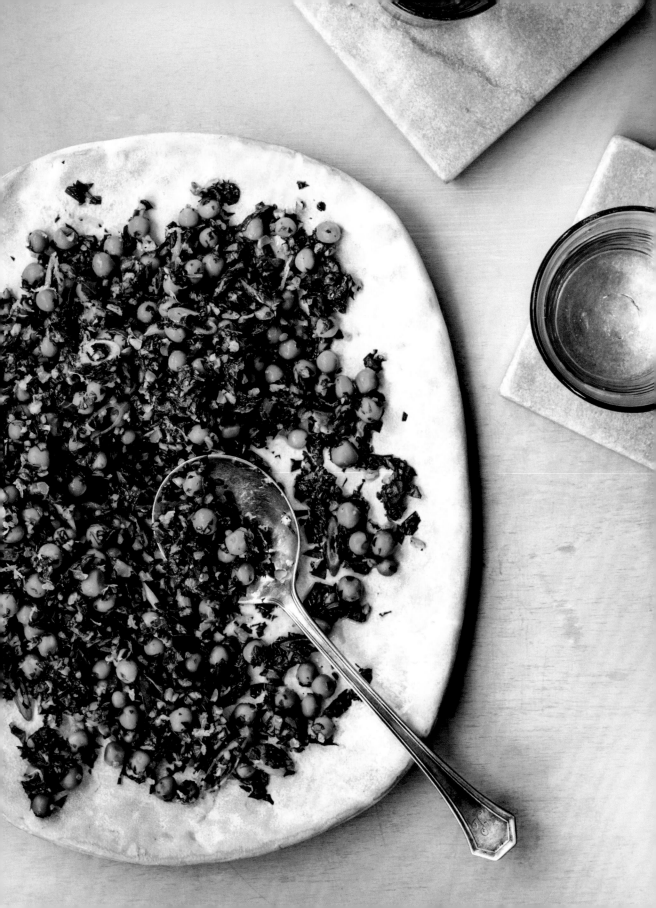

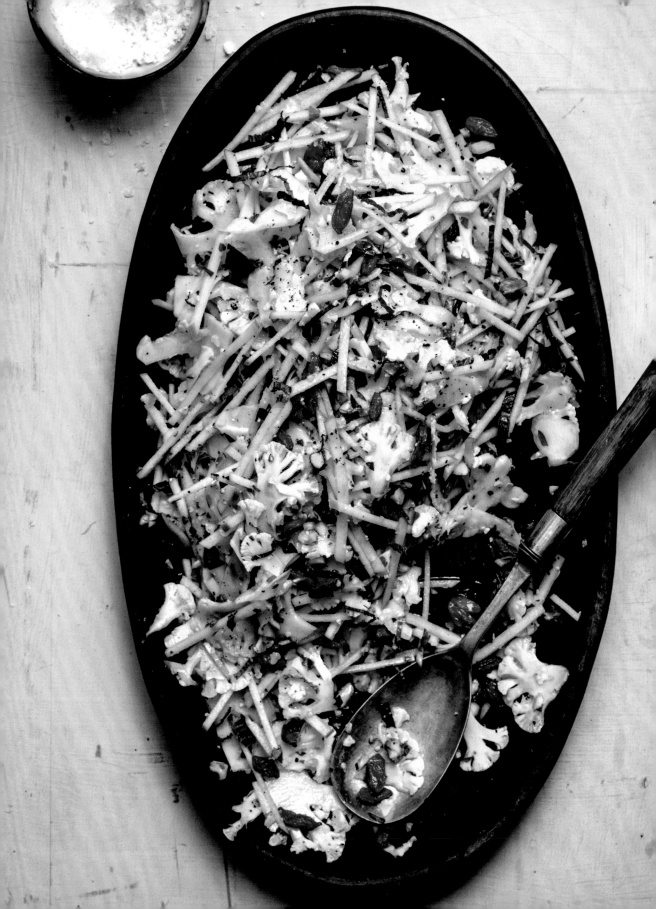

Cauliflower Salad

with Apples, Pistachios, and Goji Berries

Serves 6

1 small head **cauliflower**

2 unpeeled **Granny Smith apples**, cored and cut into matchsticks

½ cup **roasted, salted pistachios**, roughly chopped

½ cup **dried goji berries**

½ cup **fresh mint leaves**, finely chopped

½ cup **flat-leaf parsley leaves**, finely chopped

6 tablespoons **extra-virgin olive oil**

2 tablespoons **sherry vinegar**

1 tablespoon **raw honey**

1 teaspoon **Dijon mustard**

Kosher salt and freshly ground black pepper

When you shave it thin enough, there's almost no vegetable that isn't great raw. That's definitely the case with cauliflower, which brings such beautiful texture, shape, and crunch to this amazing autumn salad. It's one of Liz's all-time favorites, and it goes great with any type of protein you can throw at it—or on its own. Cauliflower is packed with vitamins, minerals, antioxidants, fiber, and choline, a nutrient we don't often get enough of that's essential for so many bodily functions. This salad keeps for days in the fridge, so go ahead and make a double batch for additional weekday meals or not-sad desk lunches.

1. With a mandoline or chef's knife, very thinly slice the cauliflower and then add it to a large bowl along with the apples, pistachios, goji berries, mint, and parsley.

2. In a small bowl, whisk together the olive oil, vinegar, honey, and mustard. Season with a pinch of salt and a twist of black pepper. Pour over the cauliflower mixture and toss together. Taste and add salt and pepper if needed. Let stand for 5 minutes before serving. Can be made a few hours in advance and stored in the fridge.

Black Bean Soup

Serves 6

1 pound **dried black beans**, soaked overnight in cold water

¼ cup **extra-virgin olive oil**

2 medium **yellow onions**, cut into ¼-inch dice

4 **garlic cloves**, minced

1 **jalapeño**, seeded and minced

Kosher salt and freshly ground black pepper

1 tablespoon **ground cumin**

2 tablespoons **ground coriander**

1 tablespoon **ground turmeric**

8 cups **Vegetable Stock**, homemade (page 240) or good-quality store-bought

½ cup **sherry vinegar**

Cilantro, for garnish

Jalapeño, for garnish

Growing up in the Midwest, I don't think I encountered a single black bean. We ate a ton of white bean soups, and we put red beans in our chili, but black bean soup just wasn't in our family rotation. It wasn't until in my late teens, when some of my cousins moved out to Texas, that I experienced my first bowl of black bean soup. Man, had I been missing out! This version is loaded with fiber and protein from the black beans and has just the right amount of heat and spice thanks to a chopped jalapeño. I like to garnish it with a few sprigs of fresh cilantro, slices of jalapeño, and a dollop of sour cream.

1. Drain and rinse the black beans and set aside.

2. Set a large saucepan over medium heat. Add the olive oil and heat to shimmering, then add the onions, garlic, minced jalapeño, and a pinch of salt. Cook until the vegetables are tender, about 5 minutes. Add the cumin, coriander, turmeric, and 2 teaspoons black pepper and cook, stirring constantly, for 1 minute. Add the stock and black beans and bring to a simmer. Cook, partially covered and stirring occasionally, until the beans are completely tender, about 1½ hours.

3. Remove the soup from the heat. Using a ladle, carefully transfer about half of the beans and liquid to a blender or food processor and puree until smooth. Stir the puree back into the soup. If it appears too thick, stir in a little water. Stir in the vinegar, taste and season with salt if needed, and serve. Garnish with cilantro and jalapeño.

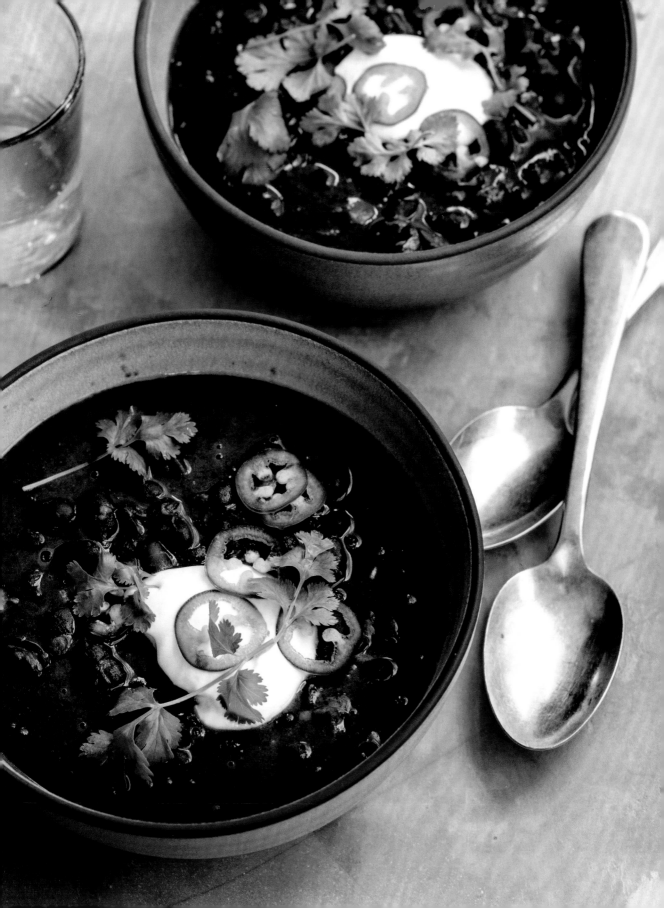

Celery Root and Chestnut Soup

Serves 6

2 cups **unshelled chestnuts** or 1 cup packed chestnut meats

2 tablespoons **extra-virgin olive oil**

1 large **yellow onion**, cut into ½–inch dice

Kosher salt and freshly ground black pepper

1 pound **celery root**, peeled and roughly chopped (about 4 cups)

1 **Granny Smith apple**, peeled, cored, and roughly chopped

4 cups **Vegetable Stock**, homemade (page 240) or good-quality store-bought

4 cups **whole milk**

2 teaspoons **freshly grated nutmeg**

1 teaspoon **ground turmeric**

1 tablespoon **apple cider vinegar**, plus more as needed

Around the holidays, whole chestnuts begin popping up in grocery stores and I'm always looking for new ways to use them because I love their sweet, nutty flavor and creamy texture once they're pureed. This elegant soup is so comforting that it's worth a little extra effort to roast and peel the chestnuts yourself (that said, some places sell roasted and peeled ones in jars or vacuum-sealed bags that make recipes like this a breeze). If you're feeling really daring, you can try roasting the chestnuts over an open fire, which adds a toasty undertone.

1. Preheat the oven to 400°F.

2. Using a sharp knife, cut a shallow X into the rounded side of each chestnut. Place them on a sheet pan and cook until the shells peel back, about 35 minutes. When cool enough to handle, remove the tough outer shell and papery skins. Roughly chop and set aside.

3. Set a large saucepan over medium heat. Add the olive oil and heat to shimmering, then add the onion and a pinch of salt. Cook until the onion begins to soften, about 2 minutes. Add the chopped chestnuts, celery root, apple, and a pinch of salt and continue cooking until the celery root begins to soften, about 5 minutes. Add the stock, milk, nutmeg, turmeric, and 1 teaspoon black pepper and bring to a simmer. Cook, partially covered, until the vegetables are very tender, about 45 minutes.

4. Remove the soup from the heat. Using a ladle, carefully transfer the soup to a blender or food processor in batches and puree until smooth. Return the soup to the saucepan and stir in the vinegar. Taste and adjust the salt, pepper, and vinegar if needed, and serve.

Yellow Squash Stew

Serves 4

3½ tablespoons **extra-virgin olive oil**

1 medium **yellow onion**, cut into 1-inch chunks

2 **garlic cloves**, minced

2 tablespoons finely chopped **fresh rosemary**

Kosher salt and freshly ground black pepper

3 **yellow squash**, cut into 1-inch chunks

1 cup roughly **chopped walnuts**

1 (28-ounce) can **crushed San Marzano tomatoes**

½ cup **Vegetable Stock**, homemade (page 240) or good-quality store-bought

2 cups **spinach leaves**

This is another great way to keep up with the fast and furious squash harvest, when they seem to appear and ripen practically overnight. I call this a stew, but it's not nearly as heavy as most and it only requires a fraction of the time to prepare. You don't often see nuts in stews, but I love the crunch and flavor (and antioxidants and "good fats") that the walnuts provide.

1. Set a large Dutch oven over medium heat. Add 3 tablespoons of the olive oil and heat to shimmering, then add the onion, garlic, rosemary, and a pinch of salt. Cook, stirring occasionally, until the onion begins to soften, about 2 minutes.

2. Add the squash, walnuts, and the remaining ½ tablespoon olive oil and cook, stirring occasionally, until the squash beings to soften, about 10 minutes. Add the tomatoes and stock, season with another pinch of salt and a twist of black pepper, and simmer until most of the liquid has evaporated and the soup has thickened, about 30 minutes. Remove from the heat, add the spinach leaves, and stir until wilted, about 1 minute. Serve.

Chickpea, Kale, and Tomato Stew

Serves 4 to 6

3 tablespoons **extra-virgin olive oil**

2 medium **yellow onions**, cut into ¼-inch dice

2 **garlic cloves**, minced

1 **jalapeño**, seeded and minced

1 tablespoon grated **fresh ginger**

Kosher salt and freshly ground black pepper

1 tablespoon **Curry Paste** (page 248) or curry powder

2 (15-ounce) cans **chickpeas**, drained and rinsed

2 cups **Vegetable Stock**, homemade (page 240) or good-quality store-bought

1 (28-ounce) can **crushed San Marzano tomatoes**

2 bunches **kale leaves and tender stems**, sliced 1-inch thick

Juice of ½ lemon

I've always liked chickpeas, but after learning about their numerous health benefits, including as a great source of manganese, a trace mineral that is a strong antioxidant and inflammation buster, I've made an effort to cook with them more. In addition to the chickpeas, this hearty stew gets a nutritional boost from heaps of kale. Know going in that kale shrinks considerably when cooked, so what might appear to be a giant bunch wilts down to just the right amount. The fresh lemon at the end really brightens up the stew.

1. Set a large Dutch oven over medium heat. Add the olive oil and heat to shimmering, then add the onions, garlic, jalapeño, ginger, and a pinch of salt. Cook, stirring occasionally, until the vegetables begin to soften, about 2 minutes. Stir in the curry paste (or powder) and cook for 30 seconds.

2. Add the chickpeas, stock, and tomatoes and bring to a simmer. Season with another pinch of salt and a twist of black pepper. Add the kale and cook, partially covered, until it's tender, about 20 minutes.

3. Remove from the heat and stir in the lemon juice. Taste and add salt and pepper if needed. Serve.

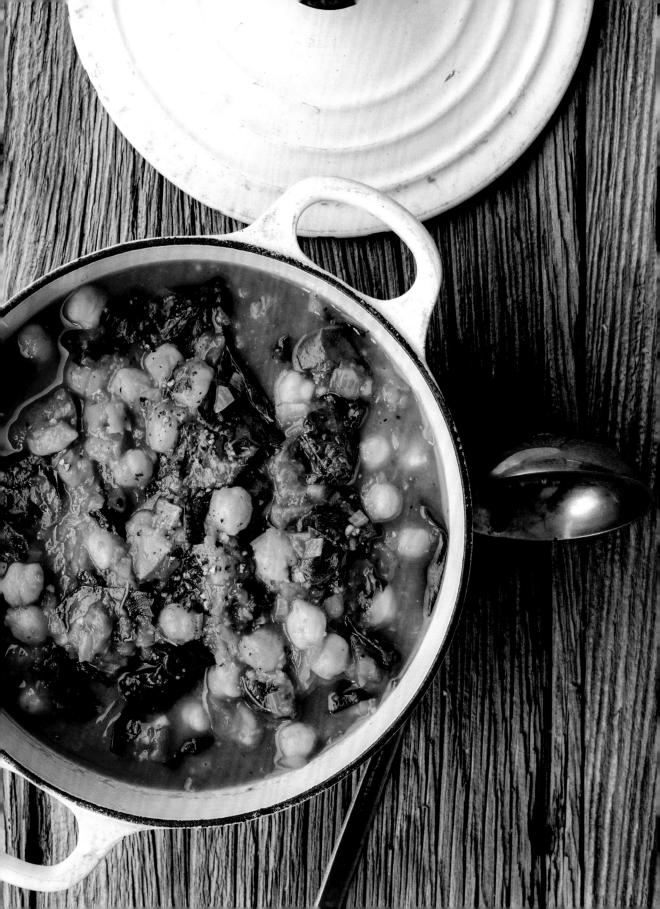

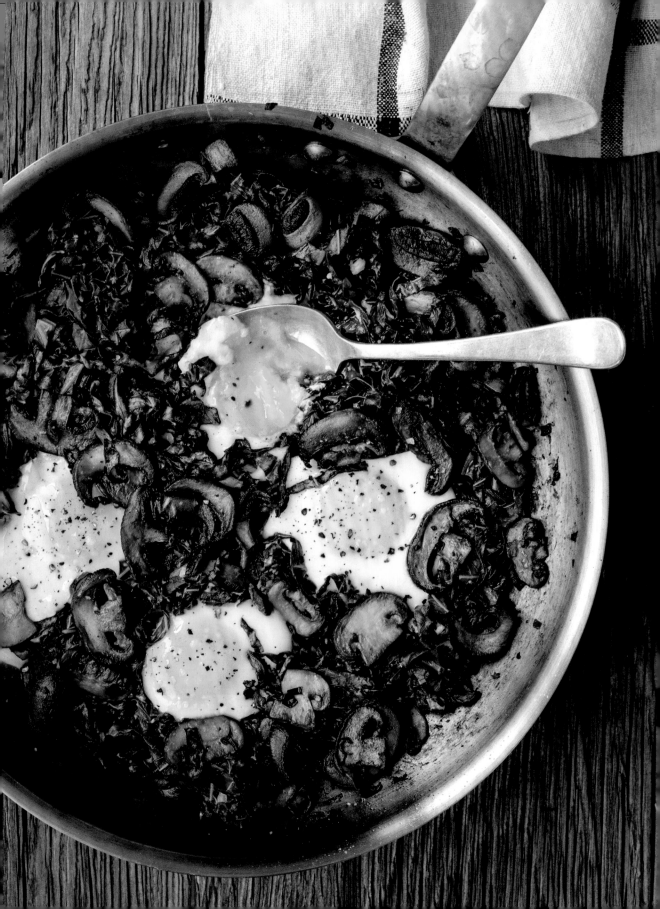

Baked Eggs

with Mushrooms, Collards, and Onions

Serves 4

3 tablespoons **extra-virgin olive oil**

1 medium **red onion**, cut into ¼-inch dice

3 cups **cremini mushrooms**, thinly sliced

Kosher salt and freshly ground black pepper

2 tablespoons **unsalted butter**

24 ounces **collard greens**, tough stems removed, thinly sliced (about 4 cups)

1 teaspoon **fresh thyme leaves**, chopped

4 large **eggs**

This is a twist on shakshuka, an Israeli dish of eggs poached in a flavorful tomato sauce. This version loads up on umami-rich mushrooms and wholesome collard greens, which are low in calories and high in vitamins, minerals, and fiber, and have remarkable detoxifying capabilities. Collards are as healthy as trendy kale but cost a fraction of the price. You can eat this one-skillet dish for breakfast, lunch, or dinner. I like to serve this with some whole-grain toast.

1. Preheat the oven to 375°F.

2. Set a large heavy-bottomed skillet over medium-high heat. Add the olive oil and heat to shimmering, then add the onion, mushrooms, and a pinch of salt. Cook until the vegetables begin to soften, about 5 minutes.

3. Add the butter, collards, and thyme and cook, stirring occasionally, until the greens are wilted and the mushrooms are golden brown, about 5 minutes. Season with another pinch of salt and a twist of black pepper.

4. Make 4 shallow depressions in the vegetable mixture and carefully crack an egg into each one. Transfer to the oven and bake until the whites are set but the yolks are still runny, about 8 minutes (or 10 if you prefer your yolks more set).

Mushroom Bolognese

Serves 4

1½ pounds **mixed wild mushrooms** (such as shiitake caps), tough stems removed

¼ cup **extra-virgin olive oil**

1 medium **yellow onion**, cut into ¼-inch dice

1 medium **carrot**, cut into ¼-inch dice

1 **celery rib**, cut into ¼-inch dice

2 **garlic cloves**, minced

Kosher salt and freshly ground black pepper

1 tablespoon **fresh thyme leaves**

3 tablespoons **tomato paste**

1 cup **whole milk**

1 pound fresh or dried **pappardelle pasta**

¼ cup **fresh basil leaves**, thinly sliced

1 cup **freshly grated parmesan cheese**, plus more for serving

Like many great inventions, this one was born out of necessity. Lizzie was craving a savory pasta dish and I was pining for my mom's classic meat sauce. By starting with a good amount of woodsy mushrooms, you begin to build up layers of meat-like flavor. Whole milk provides some body and freshly grated parmesan the nutty, salty finish. Compromise never tasted so good!

1. In a food processor, pulse the mushrooms until they have the consistency of coarse bread crumbs, about 10 times. Set aside.

2. Set a large heavy-bottomed skillet over medium-high heat. Add the olive oil and heat to shimmering, then add the onion, carrot, celery, garlic, and a pinch of salt. Cook until the vegetables begin to soften, about 5 minutes. Add the mushrooms and thyme and cook until the mushrooms begin to brown, about 5 minutes. Add the tomato paste and cook, stirring constantly, for 1 minute. Add the milk, season with another pinch of salt and a twist of black pepper, and bring to a simmer.

3. Meanwhile, add 3 tablespoons salt to a large pot of water and bring to a boil over high heat. Add the pasta and cook until just al dente, about 1 minute less than the package directions. Occasionally give the pasta a stir so it doesn't stick together. When the pasta is ready, scoop out and reserve ¼ cup of the pasta water before draining the pasta in a colander.

4. Add the pasta to the mushroom mixture along with the reserved pasta water. Remove the skillet from the heat, add the basil and parmesan, and stir to combine. Top with more freshly grated parmesan at the table.

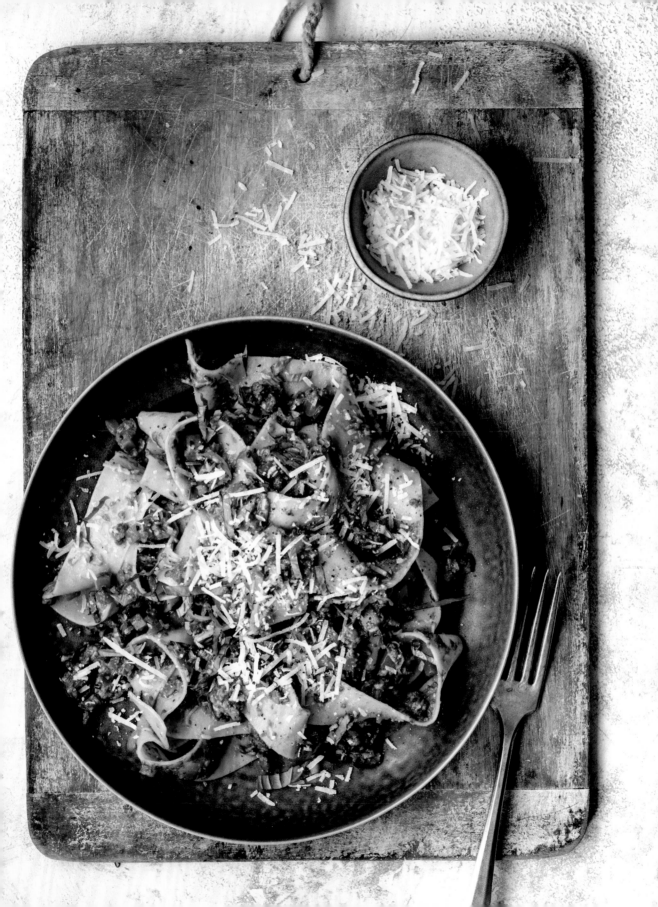

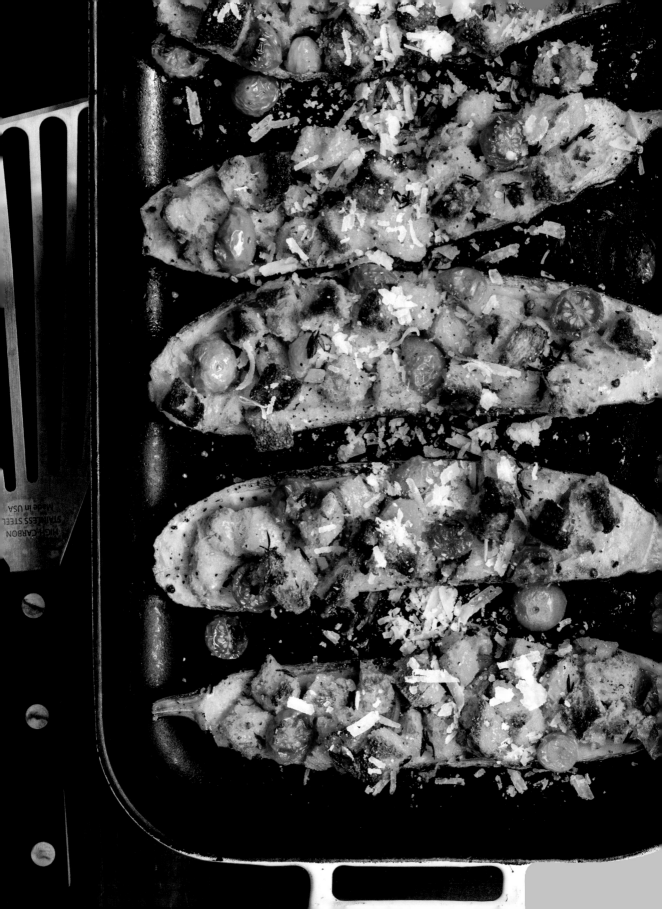

Zucchini Stuffed
with Bread Crumbs and Tomatoes

Serves 4

6 cups **sourdough bread cubes** (¼-inch)

4 medium to large **zucchini**, halved lengthwise, seeds scooped out with a spoon to form a shallow trough

6 tablespoons **extra-virgin olive oil**

Kosher salt and freshly ground black pepper

½ cup **freshly grated parmesan cheese**

2 tablespoons finely chopped **fresh thyme**

1 **garlic clove**, grated

1½ cups **Vegetable Stock**, homemade (page 240) or good-quality store-bought

1 cup **grape tomatoes**, halved

This is a great way to use zucchini that grew a little bit too fast in your garden before you got the chance to pick them. Because they're nice and big, they make perfect candidates for stuffing. I halve them and then scoop out and discard the seeds (they can be tough and bitter), replace them with a satisfying parmesan-and-tomato herbed bread crumb filling, and bake it all together. Lizzie and I love to eat these for lunch or a light dinner. Pair them with a nice salad like the Cauliflower Salad with Apples, Pistachios, and Goji Berries (page 165) to turn it into a larger meal.

1. Preheat the oven to 350°F.

2. Spread the bread cubes on a sheet pan and cook until lightly toasted, about 15 minutes. Set aside.

3. Increase the oven temperature to 450°F. Line a sheet pan with parchment paper.

4. Arrange the zucchini skin-side down on the lined sheet pan, making sure to leave some space between them. Drizzle with 3 tablespoons of the olive oil, season with a few pinches of salt and twists of black pepper, and set aside.

5. In a large bowl, stir together the remaining 3 tablespoons olive oil, the parmesan, thyme, garlic, and a pinch of salt. Add the toasted bread, stock, tomatoes, a pinch of salt, and a twist of black pepper and toss well to combine. Set aside for 15 minutes to allow the bread to absorb the liquid.

6. Divide the filling equally among the zucchini. Bake uncovered until the zucchini and the filling are cooked through, about 30 minutes. Serve hot or at room temperature.

Fresh Veggie Frittata

Serves 4

8 large **eggs**

¼ cup **plain whole-milk Greek yogurt**

Kosher salt and freshly ground black pepper

1 tablespoon **extra-virgin olive oil**

12 ounces **Swiss chard**, tough stems removed, leaves thinly sliced (about 2 cups)

1 small **zucchini**, cut into ½-inch pieces (about 1 cup)

½ cup **grape tomatoes**, quartered

¼ cup **fresh basil leaves**, thinly sliced

I'm not a huge fan of nonstick pans, because they don't produce those great crusts and flavor-developing fonds like cast-iron or aluminum-clad steel. That said, they sure do take the stress out of making a frittata! (Just make sure yours can go into the oven.) If you have access to farm-fresh eggs from pastured hens, which are sold at nearly every farmers' market and in a lot of grocery stores, too, I really think they're worth the added expense. The eggs taste better, they're higher in omega-3 fatty acids, the chickens live better lives, and you're supporting a small family farm. Now, that's what I call a win-win-win-win!

1. Preheat the broiler to high heat.

2. In a large bowl, whisk together the eggs and yogurt. Season with a pinch of salt and a twist of black pepper. Set aside.

3. Set a large ovenproof nonstick skillet over medium-high heat. Add the olive oil and heat to shimmering, then add the Swiss chard and zucchini. Season with a pinch of salt and a twist of black pepper and cook until the vegetables soften, about 3 minutes. Add the egg mixture and cook, gently stirring, until the eggs begin to set up, but are still runny, about 3 minutes. Arrange the tomatoes on top, place under the broiler, and cook until lightly golden brown, about 2 minutes.

4. Slide the frittata out of the pan onto a plate, garnish with basil, slice into wedges, and serve.

Vegetable Pot Pie

Serves 8

1 (10 × 15-inch) sheet frozen **puff pastry**, thawed

8 tablespoons (1 stick) **unsalted butter**

1 small **yellow onion**, finely chopped

1 **celery rib**, thinly sliced

Kosher salt and freshly ground black pepper

1 medium **sweet potato**, peeled and cut into ¼-inch dice

1 medium **celery root**, peeled and cut into ¼-inch dice

1 large **parsnip**, peeled and thinly sliced into rounds

1 medium **turnip**, peeled and cut into ¼-inch dice

1 tablespoon **fresh thyme leaves**, finely chopped

½ cup **unbleached, nonbromated flour**, plus more for the work surface

4 cups **Vegetable Stock**, homemade (page 240) or good-quality store-bought

½ cup finely chopped **fresh flat-leaf parsley**

If you love the comfort-food qualities of chicken pot pie—and who doesn't?—but want to go meatless, this is the way to do it. This gratifying dish has all the flavors and textures of the pot pie we love, but accomplishes it with hearty root vegetables like parsnips, turnips, and celery root. A great homemade Vegetable Stock (page 240) really comes to the rescue here, providing deep, earthy richness. Golden-brown puff pastry adds the perfect crunchy topper.

1. Preheat the oven to 425°F.

2. Set the thawed puff pastry on a lightly floured surface. Cut out 8 rounds with a 3-inch biscuit cutter, place them on a large plate or sheet pan, cover with plastic wrap, and refrigerate until needed. (Discard the remaining puff pastry or save for another purpose.)

3. Set a large Dutch oven over medium heat. Add the butter, onion, celery, and a pinch of salt and cook, stirring occasionally, until the vegetables begin to soften, about 2 minutes. Add the sweet potato, celery root, parsnip, turnip, and another pinch of salt and cook, stirring occasionally, until the root vegetables begin to soften, about 10 minutes.

4. Add the thyme and flour and cook, stirring constantly, for 1 minute. Add the stock and bring to a gentle boil, stirring to eliminate any lumps. Reduce the heat to medium-low, season with another pinch of salt and a twist of black pepper, and simmer until the vegetables are very soft and the mixture thickens, about 15 minutes. Remove from the heat and stir in the parsley.

5. Arrange eight 4-ounce ramekins on a sheet pan. Using a ladle, evenly divide the stew among the ramekins, filling them three-quarters full. Top each one with a pastry round and bake until puffy and golden brown, about 15 minutes. Remove from the oven and let sit for 5 minutes before serving.

Risotto
with Almonds, Lemon, and Parsley

Serves 4 to 6

½ cup **slivered almonds**

4 cups **Vegetable Stock**, homemade (page 240) or good-quality store-bought

5 tablespoons **unsalted butter**

1 small **yellow onion**, cut into ¼-inch dice

1 **garlic clove**, minced

Kosher salt

2 cups **Arborio rice**

1 cup **dry white wine**

1 cup **freshly grated parmesan cheese**

Grated zest of 2 lemons

½ cup finely chopped **fresh flat-leaf parsley**

When I think of risotto, my thoughts usually jump to earthy flavors like mushrooms or over-the-top versions with shaved truffle, both of which pair beautifully with the requisite fistfuls of nutty Parmigiano-Reggiano cheese. But this version is on the opposite end of the flavor spectrum thanks to sunny lemon zest, bright fresh parsley, and toasty-crunchy almonds. This dish is a hearty meal on its own, but it also works great with grilled seafood or Slow-Roasted Salmon (page 87).

1. Preheat the oven to 350°F.

2. Spread the almonds on a sheet pan and cook until lightly toasted, about 8 minutes. Set aside.

3. In a medium saucepan, warm the stock over medium-low heat. Keep warm until needed.

4. Set a large heavy-bottomed skillet over medium heat. Add 4 tablespoons of the butter, the onion, garlic, and a pinch of salt. Cook until fragrant and the vegetables begin to soften, about 2 minutes. Add the rice and cook, stirring occasionally, for 2 minutes. Add the wine and cook, stirring constantly, until all of the liquid has been absorbed, about 1 minute.

5. Add 1 ladleful of the warm stock and stir constantly until most of the liquid has been absorbed. Repeat this process until all but about 1 cup of the stock has been incorporated and the rice is very creamy (and somewhat runny), but still slightly al dente, about 25 minutes. If you prefer softer rice, add the last ladleful of stock and continue to cook until the rice is done to your preference.

6. Remove the pan from the heat, stir in the remaining 1 tablespoon butter, the toasted almonds, parmesan, lemon zest, and parsley and serve immediately while the texture is still slightly runny.

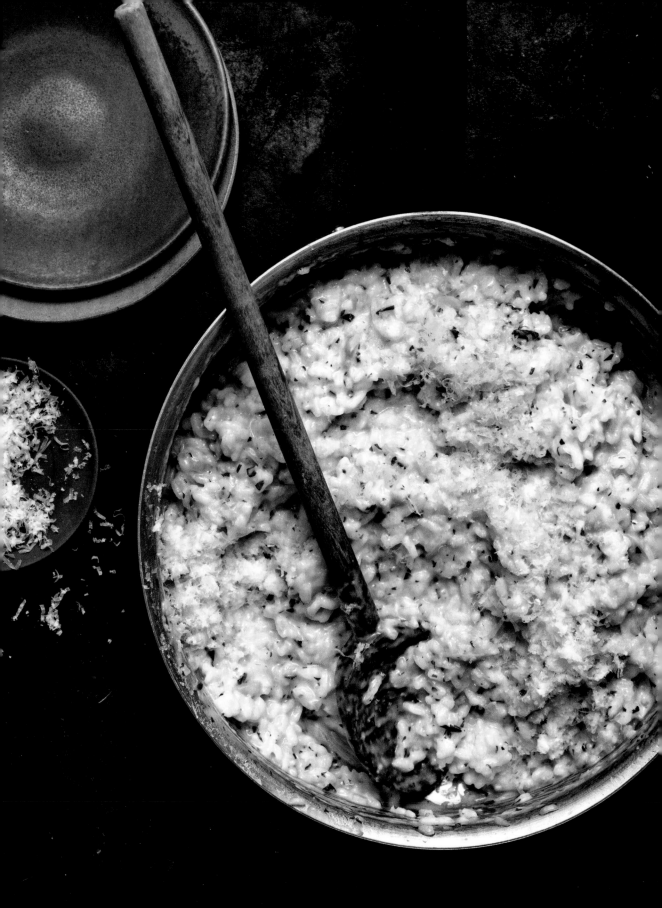

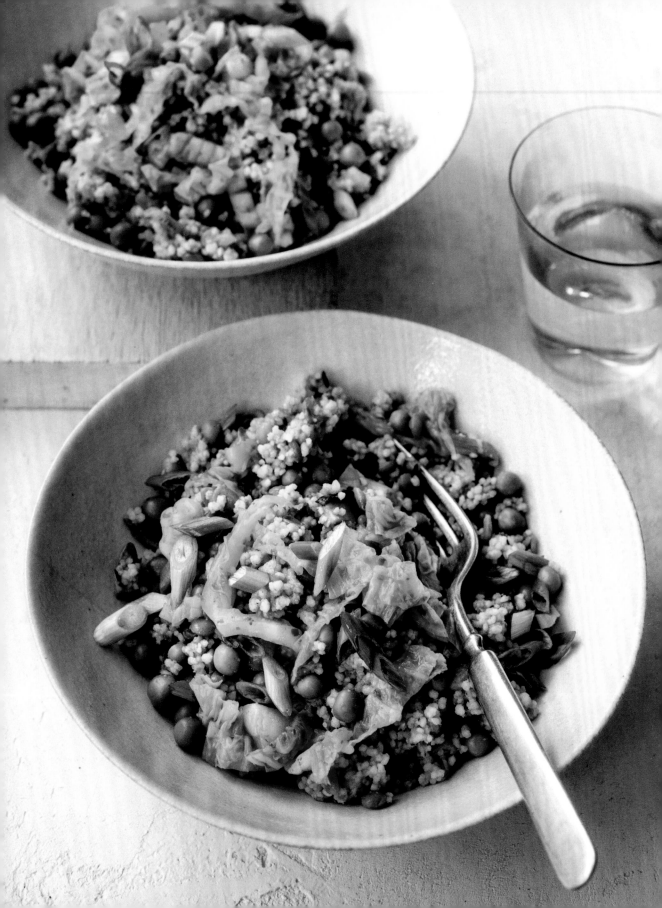

Couscous

with Lentils, Kimchi, Peas, and Mushrooms

Serves 6

2 tablespoons **extra-virgin olive oil**

1 small **yellow onion**, cut into ¼-inch dice

2 **garlic cloves**, minced

3 cups **shiitake mushrooms**, tough stems removed, thinly sliced

2 tablespoons **thyme leaves**

Kosher salt and freshly ground black pepper

4 cups **Mushroom Stock** (page 241) or good-quality store-bought

½ cup **brown lentils**, rinsed

1 cup **couscous**

2 cups fresh or frozen **shelled peas** (thawed if frozen)

4 **scallions**, thinly sliced

1 cup chopped **kimchi**

Kimchi is like the Korean version of sauerkraut, so naturally I love it! It's saltier and spicier than traditional sauerkraut, but it is every bit as crunchy, which brings great texture to this couscous dish. It has gotten so much easier to find kimchi in regular grocery stores, but if you have any Asian markets nearby, I'd start there. They typically stock many different varieties, and they're often homemade. The lentils in this grain bowl bring extra protein and fiber to the table, making it a perfect and complete meal.

1. Set a large Dutch oven over medium heat. Add the olive oil and heat to shimmering, then add the onion, garlic, mushrooms, and thyme. Cook, stirring occasionally, until the vegetables soften and begin to brown, about 5 minutes. Season with a pinch of salt and a twist of black pepper.

2. Add the stock and lentils, stir, and bring to a strong simmer. Cook, partially covered, until the lentils are tender, about 45 minutes.

3. In a large bowl, combine the couscous and peas. When the lentils are tender, pour them and any remaining cooking liquid over the couscous, stir, and cover with plastic wrap, steaming the couscous until it has absorbed the liquid and is plump and cooked, about 10 minutes.

4. Fluff the couscous with a fork, stir in the scallions and kimchi, and serve.

Tomato Gratin

Serves 4 to 6

6 large **beefsteak tomatoes**, cut into slices ¾ inch thick

2 tablespoons **extra-virgin olive oil**

Kosher salt and freshly ground black pepper

1 small **yellow onion**, very thinly sliced into rings

4 tablespoons **unsalted butter**

2 **garlic cloves**, minced

2 tablespoons finely chopped **rosemary**

¼ cup **unbleached, nonbromated flour**

2 cups **whole milk**

½ teaspoon **freshly grated nutmeg**

½ cup **mascarpone cheese**

½ cup **freshly grated parmesan cheese**

In the middle of winter, when all you want to do is hibernate in front of the fire with a glass of red wine, consider making this dish. It's almost like a tomato fondue it's so rich, cheesy, and comforting. Although oven-roasting the tomatoes might seem like a needless extra step, it's worth the trouble.

1. Preheat the oven to 300°F. Line 2 sheet pans with parchment paper.

2. Arrange the tomatoes in a single layer on the lined pans, making sure to leave some space between them. Drizzle the tomatoes with the olive oil, season with a few pinches of salt and twists of black pepper, and cook for 2 hours.

3. Increase the oven temperature to 400°F.

4. In a 9 × 13-inch baking dish, alternately arrange the tomato and onion slices in an even layer across the bottom, slightly overlapping them if necessary. Set aside.

5. Set a medium saucepan over medium heat. Add the butter, garlic, rosemary, and a pinch of salt. Cook, stirring occasionally, until the garlic is fragrant, about 1 minute. Add the flour and stir constantly until the roux is lightly golden, about 2 minutes. Whisk in the milk a little at a time to avoid lumps. Whisk in the nutmeg. Bring to a simmer and cook, stirring occasionally, for 20 minutes. Remove from the heat and whisk in the mascarpone. Season with a pinch of salt and a twist of black pepper.

6. Lightly season the tomatoes and onions with salt and pepper. Pour the sauce over the tomatoes, top evenly with the parmesan, and bake, uncovered, until the onions are tender and the cheese is golden brown, about 35 minutes. Remove from the oven and let stand for 10 minutes before serving.

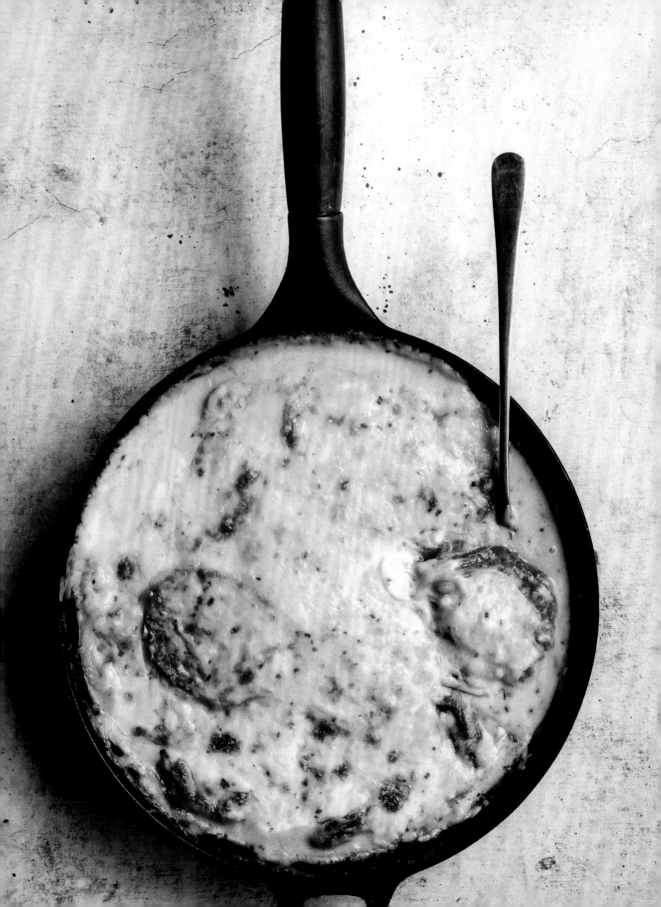

Polenta with Pomodoro

Serves 6

6 cups **chicken stock**, homemade or good-quality store-bought

5 tablespoons **extra-virgin olive oil**, plus more for drizzling

Kosher salt and freshly ground black pepper

2 cups **coarse cornmeal**

½ cup **mascarpone cheese**, plus more for garnish

⅓ cup **freshly grated parmesan cheese**

Pomodoro Sauce (page 131), warmed, or 3 cups of your favorite store-bought marinara

Polenta, which is made from corn so it's wheat-free, is such a versatile food. You can enjoy it straight out of the saucepan when it's all warm, soft, and velvety. Or you can spread it out in a pan, allow it to cool, and then cut it into firmed-up pieces and use them in all sorts of delicious ways. Here, I fry them up in a pan until crisp and fragrant. The corny polenta pairs perfectly with sweet tomato sauce and a heaping spoonful of luscious mascarpone. Fried polenta also makes a great base for recipes like Chickpea, Kale, and Tomato Stew (page 170).

1. In a large saucepan, combine the stock, 3 tablespoons of the olive oil, and 2 teaspoons salt and bring to a boil over medium-high heat. Slowly sprinkle the cornmeal into the pot, whisking constantly, until fully incorporated. Reduce the heat to low and simmer, stirring occasionally, until smooth and creamy, about 45 minutes. Add the mascarpone and parmesan and stir to combine. Taste and add salt and pepper if needed.

2. Line a 9 × 13-inch baking pan with plastic wrap. Pour in the warm polenta and use a rubber spatula to smooth it into an even layer. Refrigerate uncovered until firm, at least 2 hours or overnight.

3. Turn the polenta out onto a work surface by flipping the baking pan. Remove the plastic wrap and cut 12 equal squares.

4. Set a large heavy-bottomed skillet over medium heat. Add 1 tablespoon of the olive oil and heat to shimmering. In batches, fry the polenta squares until crisp and golden brown on both sides, about 3 minutes per side. If the pan seems dry, add the remaining 1 tablespoon olive oil.

5. Ladle some warm pomodoro sauce on a plate and top with the hot, crispy polenta. Garnish with a dollop of mascarpone, drizzle with olive oil, and serve.

Vegetable Jambalaya

Serves 6

2 tablespoons **extra-virgin olive oil**

1 large **yellow onion**, cut into ¼-inch dice

3 **celery ribs**, thinly sliced

1 **green bell pepper**, cut into ¼-inch dice

1 **jalapeño**, seeded and minced

4 **garlic cloves**, minced

Kosher salt and freshly ground black pepper

2 **fresh bay leaves**

1 tablespoon **thyme leaves**, finely chopped

1 tablespoon **smoked paprika**

2 cups brown **basmati rice**

4 cups **Vegetable Stock**, homemade (page 240) or good-quality store-bought

1 (15-ounce) can **black beans**, drained and rinsed

1 (14.5- to 15-ounce) can **crushed San Marzano tomatoes**

2 tablespoons **Worcestershire sauce**

Hot sauce

¼ cup finely chopped **fresh cilantro**

6 **lime wedges**

Jambalaya traditionally has meats like ham, andouille sausage, chicken, and even rabbit, but when Lizzie requested a vegetarian version, I was happy to oblige. This recipe has all the classic elements of a great jambalaya—smoky, spicy, and sweet—tied together by moist, flavorful rice, just none of the meat. With enough hot sauce, all things are possible!

1. Set a large Dutch oven over medium-high heat. Add the olive oil and heat to shimmering, then add the onion, celery, bell pepper, jalapeño, garlic, and a large pinch of salt. Cook, stirring occasionally, until the vegetables begin to soften, about 3 minutes.

2. Add the bay leaves, thyme, and smoked paprika and cook until the spices are toasted, about 30 seconds. Add the rice, stir constantly for 30 seconds, then add the stock, black beans, tomatoes, Worcestershire, and hot sauce to taste. Season with another pinch of salt and a twist of black pepper. Bring to a boil, reduce the heat to medium-low, cover, and simmer until the rice is tender and absorbs all of the liquid, about 1 hour.

3. Remove the pot from the heat and let stand for 5 minutes before fluffing the rice with a fork. Garnish with cilantro and serve with lime wedges and hot sauce on the side.

Sugar-Free Fix

I don't consume much added sugar in my diet. You won't find me sitting down to a bowl of "fruity" breakfast cereal, or buying packaged products that are loaded with hidden sugar (I'm looking at you, ketchup, jarred pasta sauce, and white sandwich bread). So it was surprising to me to experience the discomfort that followed the consumption of sugar while I was going through the process of identifying my triggers. No question about it: Sugar kicks my arthritis into high gear, blowing away dairy in terms of my most detrimental foods.

But that was just the beginning of my discovery. After a little more experimentation, I determined that it wasn't all sugars that caused inflammation and pain, but largely refined white sugar and ultraprocessed sweeteners like high fructose corn syrup. Interestingly, all-natural products like honey and maple syrup did not cause inflammation and all of the painful side effects that come with it. I also learned that natural sweeteners like agave, coconut sugar, and palm sugars do not adversely affect me the way highly processed granulated sugar does. (Your own personal results may vary.)

When shopping for honey and maple syrup, it's important to know what to look for and how to read the label. Many bottles of "honey" and "maple syrup" are little more than a cocktail of corn syrup and water mixed with artificial flavors and colors and a splash of preservatives. In the case of honey, look for labels that say "raw," typically meaning that it went through little more than light filtering to eliminate wax particles, air bubbles, and "bee parts." The term also usually implies that the honey is not heat-pasteurized, a process that strips away beneficial enzymes.

Like honey, maple syrup is a natural food product that is labeled and sold according to color, from pale golden to dark brown. But the color has absolutely nothing to do with quality, as all are made exactly the same way—by boiling down the sweet sap to evaporate much of the water and concentrate the sugar to make maple syrup. For most uses, I find that the amber varieties possess the perfect blend of sweet, nutty, and woodsy flavors. But beware of products that don't contain phrases like "100 percent pure maple syrup," and especially those that go by vague and misleading names like "maple-flavored syrup," "pancake syrup," or "breakfast syrup," most of which contain corn syrup and zero real maple syrup.

Yes, good-quality honey and maple syrup are not cheap, but the amounts used are relatively modest, the flavors incredibly richer and more complex, and they both store well (honey indefinitely; maple syrup for months in the fridge). When it comes to purchasing, my first stop is always the local farmers' market, where I'm typically buying it straight from the producer.

These recipes might skip the processed sugar, but they don't skimp on sweet-tooth satisfaction.

Gluten-Free Chocolate Chip Cookies

Makes 16 cookies

2 cups **almond flour**

½ teaspoon **baking soda**

½ teaspoon **kosher salt**

2 tablespoons **unsalted butter**, at room temperature

¼ cup **raw honey**

1 large **egg**

2 tablespoons **heavy cream**

2 teaspoons **vanilla extract**

½ cup **bittersweet chocolate chips**

My main goal when devising this recipe was to create a chocolate chip cookie that tasted as good as or even *better* than the ones I used to enjoy as a kid. And let me tell you, if I was anywhere near a batch of homemade chocolate chip cookies, you needed to watch out! These ones nail my cookie requirements: crisp around the edges, soft and fluffy in the middle. Plus, since they are made with almond flour rather than wheat flour, I can plow through the whole batch and feel fine. (Well, except for the guilt and shame that come with it.)

1. In a medium bowl, whisk together the almond flour, baking soda, and salt.

2. In a large bowl, whisk together the butter and honey. Whisk in the egg, cream, and vanilla. With a wooden spoon stir in the flour mixture to combine. Fold in the chocolate chips. Cover the bowl with plastic wrap and refrigerate for at least 2 hours or up to overnight.

3. Preheat the oven to 350°F. Line a sheet pan with a silicone baking mat or parchment paper.

4. Using a 1-ounce scoop, portion the cookies out onto the prepared sheet pan (you should get sixteen 2-inch balls). Slightly flatten the balls with the palms of your hands.

5. Bake the cookies until they are golden brown around the edges and puffed in the middle, about 15 minutes. Remove from the oven and let rest on the pan for 5 minutes before transferring to a cooling rack to cool completely. Store in an airtight container for up to 3 days.

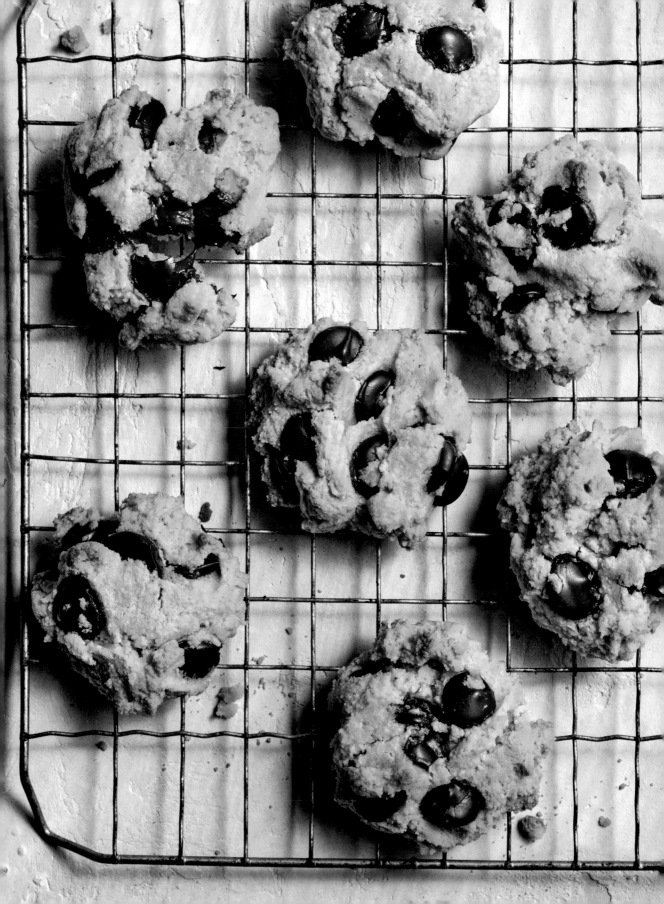

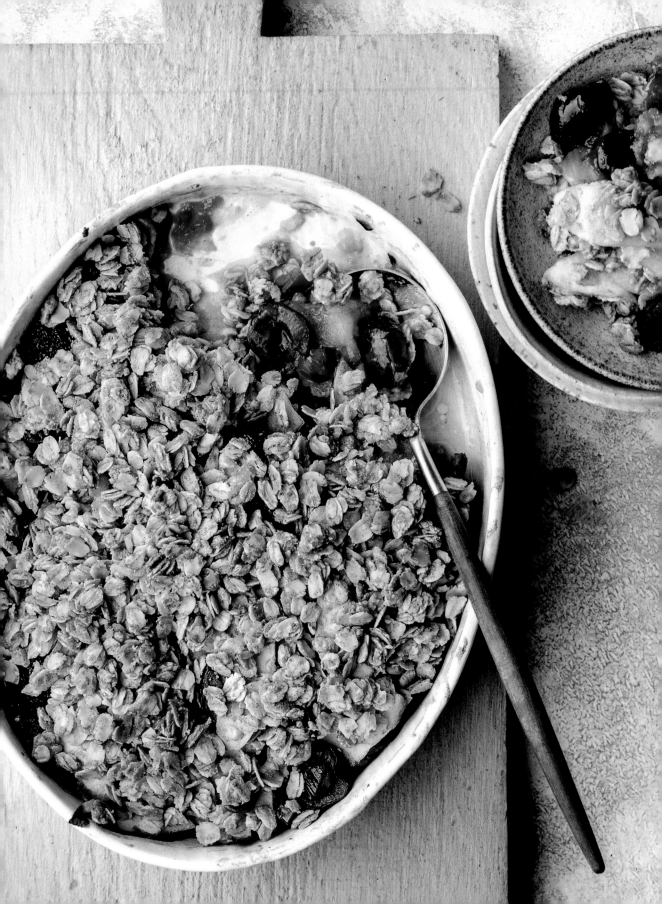

Apple-and-Cherry Oat Crisp

Serves 6

One of the benefits of baking without sugar is that it's easier to showcase the natural flavors of fruit. If it's cherry season, you definitely want to go the fresh route, but frozen fruit is remarkably versatile. I like to use great local honey with this because it pairs beautifully with the dates, but maple syrup is great, too. If you have any left over, top it with some thick and creamy yogurt and enjoy it for breakfast!

Apples and Cherries

5 **Granny Smith apples**, peeled, cored, and cut into ⅛-inch-thick slices

1 cup roughly chopped pitted **Medjool dates**

2 cups fresh or frozen **cherries**, pitted

2 tablespoons **fresh lemon juice**

½ teaspoon **kosher salt**

3 tablespoons **unsalted butter**

Topping

2 cups **old-fashioned rolled oats**

½ cup **unbleached, nonbromated flour**

1 teaspoon **ground cinnamon**

¼ teaspoon **kosher salt**

5 tablespoons **unsalted butter**, melted

2 tablespoons **pure maple syrup** or **raw honey**

1. Preheat the oven to 350°F.

2. **Prepare the apples and cherries:** In a large bowl, toss together the apples, dates, cherries, lemon juice, and salt. Spread evenly in a 9 × 13-inch baking dish. Cut the butter into 6 pieces and evenly distribute over the top.

3. **Make the topping:** In a large bowl, stir together the oats, flour, cinnamon, and salt. Drizzle in the melted butter and maple syrup and stir well to combine.

4. Sprinkle the topping evenly over the surface of the fruit mixture and bake uncovered until the apples are soft and the topping is golden brown and crisp, about 45 minutes. Serve hot or at room temperature. Store covered, unrefrigerated, for up to 2 days.

Blueberries and Cream Paleta

with Mint

Makes 10 freezer pops

2 cups **blueberries**

½ cup **fresh mint leaves**

2 tablespoons **agave nectar**

Grated zest of ½ lime

¼ cup **fresh lime juice** (from about 1 lime)

¼ cup **crème fraîche**

Pinch of **kosher salt**

My mom used to make homemade frozen pops for us with whatever fruit happened to be lying around. If you've never had a blueberry and mint version, you're totally missing out. To simplify things, you can purchase awesome molds for about $10, but small paper cups and even ice cube trays also work. Another route you could take is to pour the liquid mixture into a baking dish, freeze it, and scrape it into refreshing granita.

1. In a blender or food processor, combine ¾ cup water, the blueberries, mint, agave, lime zest, lime juice, crème fraîche, and salt and process until completely smooth, about 1 minute.

2. Pour evenly into ten 3-ounce ice pop molds and freeze, until hard and set, at least 4 hours and up to overnight.

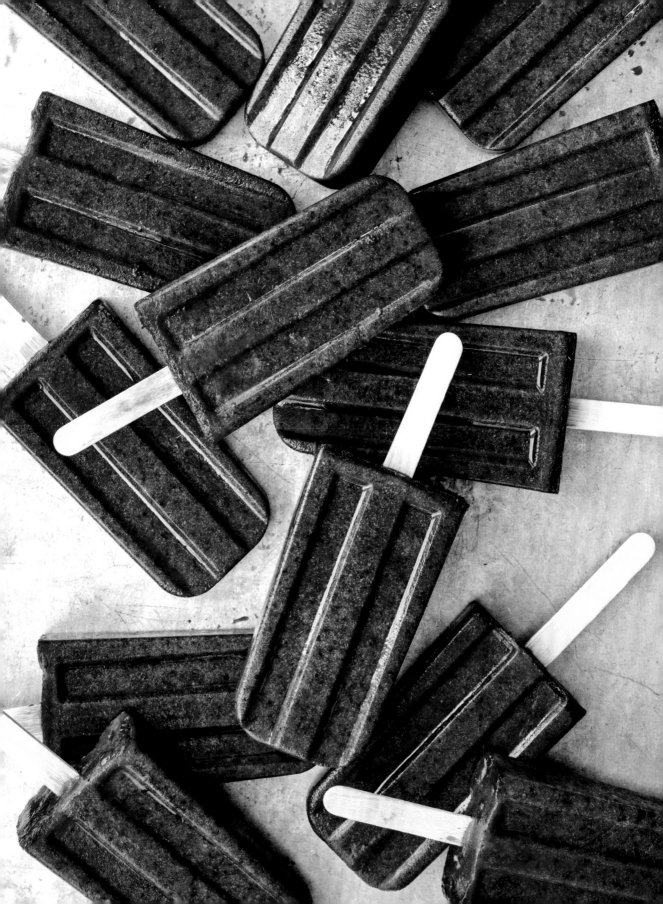

Lemon-Orange Bars

**Makes twenty-four
2-inch squares**

12 tablespoons (1½ sticks) **unsalted butter**, at room temperature

2 tablespoons **raw honey**

2⅓ cups **unbleached, nonbromated flour**

¼ teaspoon **kosher salt**

6 large **eggs**

¾ cup **heavy cream**

¾ cup **raw honey**

Grated zest and juice of 2 oranges

½ cup **fresh lemon juice** (about 2 lemons)

Lemon bars were all the rage growing up, and every household seemed to have its own recipe. But all of them tended to offer the same sweet-tart punch that was simultaneously too sweet and too tart. This version is more understated, thanks to the addition of orange juice to tone down the pucker from the lemon and honey in place of all that granulated sugar. Make an extra batch to share with the neighbors—they'll thank you!

1. Preheat the oven to 350°F.

2. In a stand mixer fitted with the paddle, cream the butter and honey on medium speed until smooth, about 1 minute. Add 2 cups of the flour and the salt and mix on medium speed until coarse crumbs form, about 1 minute. Press the mixture evenly into the bottom of a 9 × 13-inch baking pan and bake until light golden brown, about 20 minutes. Remove from the oven and set aside. Leave the oven on.

3. In a stand mixer fitted with the whisk, whip the eggs, cream, honey, the remaining ⅓ cup flour, and the orange zest on medium speed until smooth. With the mixer running on low, slowly add the orange juice and lemon juice and continue to beat on medium speed until just combined, about 1 minute.

4. Pour the batter onto the crust and bake until light golden brown, about 30 minutes. Remove from the oven and allow to cool slightly. While still warm, slice into 24 squares and allow to cool to room temperature. Cover the pan with plastic wrap and refrigerate until cold, at least 2 hours or up to overnight. Store for up to 3 days covered in the fridge.

Gluten-Free Chocolate-Glazed Doughnuts

**Makes twelve
3-inch doughnuts**

I should probably win some kind of award for coming up with a granulated sugar–free, gluten-free chocolate doughnut that is this delicious. The rich chocolate flavor really shines through, and the cake-based doughnut is so delicate that it melts in your mouth. These gems even earned the approval of Kyle, the brains behind Grindstone Coffee & Donuts in Sag Harbor, New York, and a doughnut purist if ever there was one. Who knows, maybe he'll even find some rack space at the shop for them one day!

Doughnuts

2 ounces **dark (70% cacao or higher) chocolate**, roughly chopped

3 tablespoons **unsalted butter**

3 tablespoons **coconut oil**

2 cups **almond flour**

3 tablespoons **unsweetened cocoa powder**

1 teaspoon **baking powder**

½ teaspoon **baking soda**

½ teaspoon **kosher salt**

¼ teaspoon **espresso powder**

2 large **eggs**

¼ cup **pure maple syrup**

¼ cup **heavy cream**

1 teaspoon **vanilla extract**

Ganache

2 ounces **(70% cacao or higher) dark chocolate**, chopped

¼ cup **heavy cream**

1. Preheat the oven to 350°F. Grease a 12-doughnut pan or two 6-doughnut pans with cooking spray.

2. **Make the doughnuts:** In a saucepan, bring 1 inch water to a boil over high heat. Reduce the heat to low, set a heatproof bowl over the saucepan (make sure the bottom of the bowl doesn't touch the hot water), and add the chocolate, butter, and coconut oil. Stir until completely melted and smooth, about 3 minutes. Remove from the heat and set aside to cool.

3. In a large bowl, whisk to combine the almond flour, cocoa powder, baking powder, baking soda, salt, and espresso powder.

4. In a separate large bowl, whisk together the eggs, maple syrup, cream, and vanilla. Add the chocolate mixture and whisk to combine. Add the dry ingredients and stir with a rubber spatula to combine.

5. Divide the batter among the doughnut molds, filling each halfway full. Bake until the doughnuts are puffed and beginning to crack, about 12 minutes. Remove the pan from the oven and set aside to cool for about 5 minutes. When the pan is cool enough to handle, turn the doughnuts out onto a cooling rack while you make the ganache.

▶ Recipe continues

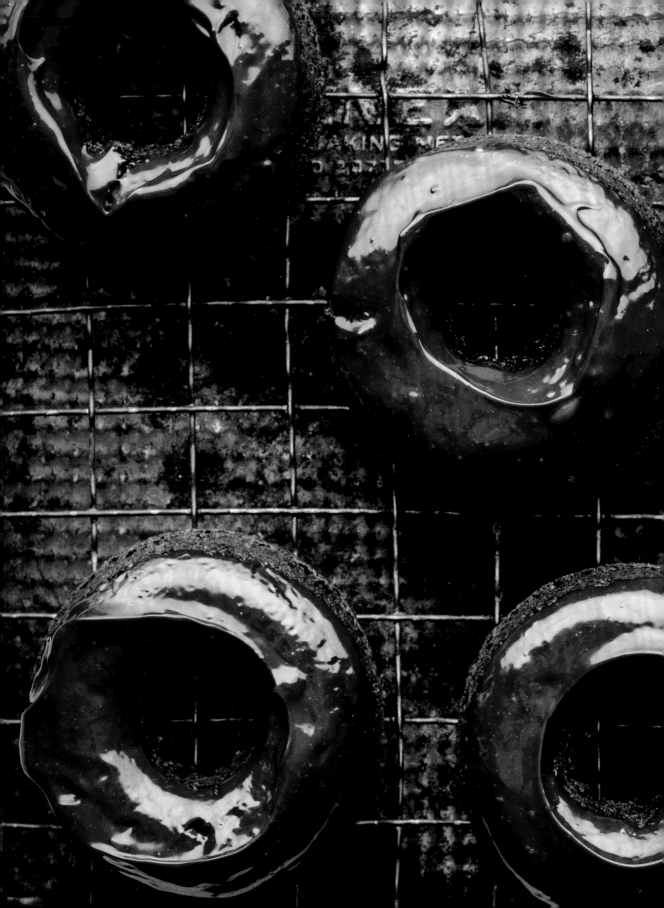

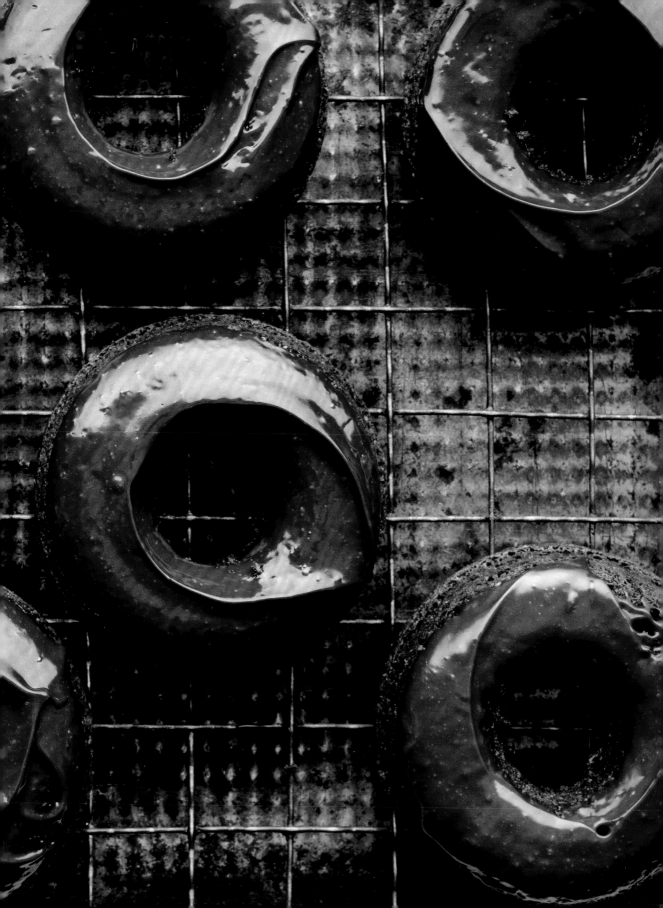

6. **Make the ganache:** Place the dark chocolate in a heatproof bowl. In a small saucepan, bring the cream to a strong simmer over medium-high heat. Pour the hot cream over the chocolate and set aside for 3 minutes to melt. Whisk until the mixture is completely smooth and then let it stand at room temperature for 20 minutes to slightly thicken.

7. Dip the top half of each doughnut into the ganache and place on the cooling rack to drip and set. These doughnuts are best when really fresh, but they keep overnight stored in an airtight container.

Gluten-Free Peanut Butter, Oatmeal, and Banana Cookies

Makes 26 cookies

2 large ripe **bananas**, mashed

2 large **eggs**

1 cup **natural creamy peanut butter**

3 tablespoons **raw honey**

3 tablespoons **pure maple syrup**

1 teaspoon **vanilla extract**

2½ cups **old-fashioned rolled oats**

1 teaspoon **ground cinnamon**

½ teaspoon **kosher salt**

When I end up with a couple of really ripe bananas, I often make these cookies, which provide all the pleasure and little of the guilt of bakery-bought varieties. In addition to peanut butter and banana being one of the world's all-time best flavor combos, the fruit helps keep these cookies moist and soft. A lot of natural foods stores and even regular grocers now have stations where you can grind your own nut butters. The freshness and flavor can't be beat, there are no added ingredients like hydrogenated oil (trans fat) and sugar, and they actually cost less than prepackaged name brands. Keep all fresh-ground nut butters in the fridge where they'll stay their freshest. And did I mention these are gluten-free?!

1. In a medium bowl, stir together the mashed banana and eggs. Add the peanut butter, honey, maple syrup, and vanilla and stir to combine. Add the oats, cinnamon, and salt and stir to combine. Cover the bowl with plastic wrap and refrigerate until the batter is cold and not very sticky, at least 3 hours or up to overnight.

2. Preheat the oven to 350°F. Line two sheet pans with a silicone baking mat.

3. Using a 1-ounce scoop, portion the cookies out onto the prepared sheet pan. Slightly flatten the balls with the palms of your hands. Bake the cookies until they are golden brown and set, about 15 minutes. Remove from the oven and let rest on the pan for 5 minutes before transferring to a cooling rack to cool completely. Store in an airtight container at room temperature for up to 3 days.

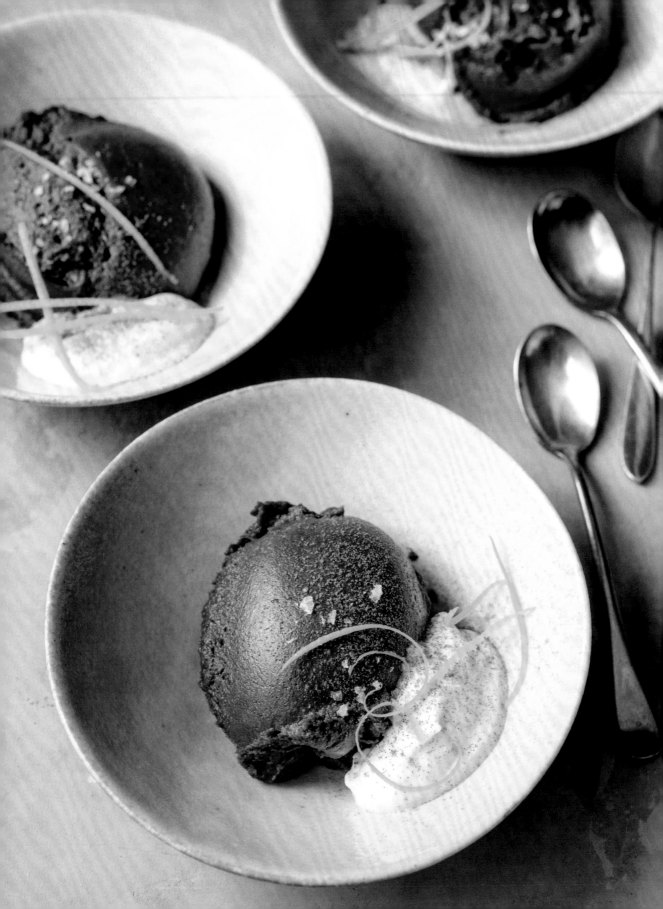

Chocolate Mousse

Serves 6

2 large **avocados**, diced

1 cup **coconut cream** (not cream of coconut)

¼ cup **unsweetened cocoa powder**

¼ cup fresh **orange juice**

¼ cup **raw honey** or **pure maple syrup**

1 teaspoon **vanilla extract**

¾ teaspoon **ground cinnamon**

Kosher salt

I know it's probably strange to see avocado in a dessert recipe, but it's the secret ingredient to a delectable dairy-free mousse with silky texture—it also gives the mousse an extra dose of potassium. When shopping for coconut cream, make sure you don't accidentally grab cream of coconut, coconut milk, or coconut water, which are entirely different products. Coconut cream is rich, thick, and (duh) creamy, and it's essential to getting the best results. If you can't find coconut cream, you can scoop out the cream that rises to the top of an unshaken can of coconut milk. You'll probably need two or three cans' worth.

1. In a stand mixer fitted with the whisk, combine the avocados, coconut cream, and cocoa powder. Mix on low until combined and then slowly increase the speed to medium until completely smooth and aerated, about 2 minutes.

2. Add the orange juice, honey, vanilla, cinnamon, and a pinch of salt and mix on low until combined, about 30 seconds. Increase the speed to high and blend for 1 minute.

3. Cover the bowl with plastic wrap and chill for at least 2 hours or up to overnight before serving.

Gluten-Free Chocolate-Pecan Cake

with Ganache

Makes one 8-inch cake

This recipe is a little bit more involved than others, but the results are worth it—especially for those in search of a decadent chocolate cake that also happens to be gluten-free. The avocado adds creaminess and body to the cake, the honey and maple syrup provide subtle, natural sweetness, and the toasted pecans bring a pleasant crunch to the party. Just before serving, I like to sprinkle a little flaky sea salt on top for added texture. To make this cake dairy-free, substitute full-fat coconut milk for the heavy cream in the ganache.

Cake

1 cup **pecan halves**

¾ cup **coconut flour**

¾ cup **tapioca flour**

2 teaspoons **baking soda**

2 tablespoons **cocoa powder**

1 teaspoon **instant espresso powder**

¾ teaspoon **sea salt**

1½ cups diced **avocado** (about 2 avocados)

4 large **eggs**, separated

¾ cup **raw honey**

2 tablespoons **pure maple syrup**

1 tablespoon **vanilla extract**

4 ounces **dark (70% cacao or higher) chocolate**, melted and cooled

2 tablespoons **coconut oil**, melted

Ganache

2 ounces **dark (70% cacao or higher) chocolate**, chopped

¼ cup **heavy cream**

1. Preheat the oven to 350°F.

2. **Make the cake:** Spread the pecans on a sheet pan and cook until lightly toasted, about 8 minutes. Remove from the oven and set aside to cool. Once cool enough to handle, roughly chop and set aside.

3. Leave the oven on. Cut a piece of parchment paper to fit the bottom of an 8-inch round cake pan. Coat the inside of the pan and the parchment paper with cooking spray.

4. In a medium bowl, whisk together the coconut flour, tapioca flour, baking soda, cocoa powder, espresso powder, and sea salt.

5. In a stand mixer fitted with the paddle, cream together the avocado, egg yolks, honey, maple syrup, and vanilla on medium speed until well combined and smooth, about 2 minutes. Add the melted chocolate and coconut oil and mix until just combined. Add the dry ingredients and mix until just combined. Transfer the batter to a large bowl and set aside. Clean out the mixer bowl.

6. In the clean bowl of the stand mixer fitted with the whisk, beat the egg whites to soft peaks. Gently fold

▶ Recipe continues

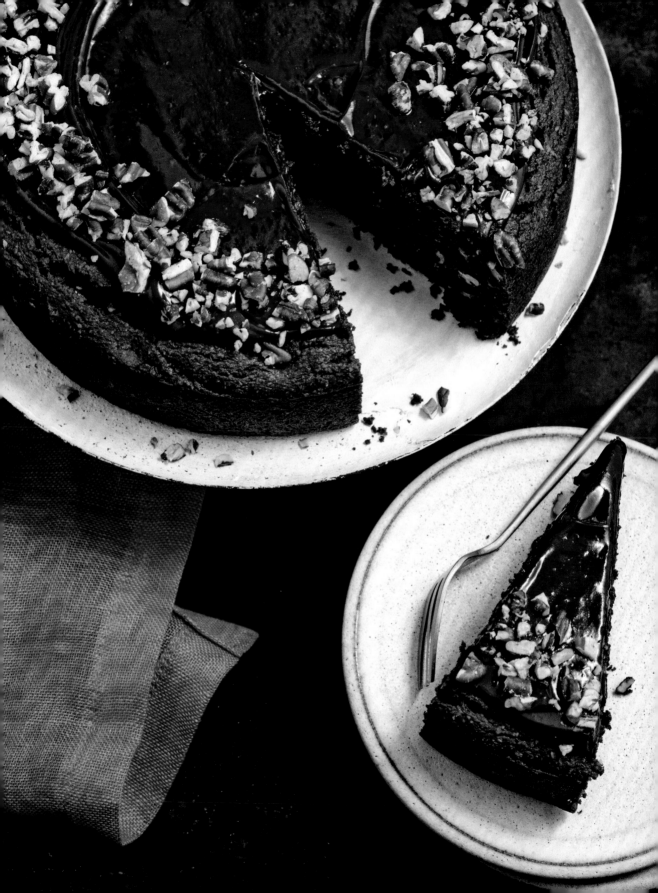

the beaten whites into the cake batter in two separate batches until no white streaks remain. Gently fold in ¾ cup of the chopped pecans.

7. Pour the batter into the prepared pan and smooth the top. Bake until a toothpick inserted into the center comes out clean, about 40 minutes. Remove the cake from the oven and set aside to cool completely in the pan, at least 1 hour or up to overnight.

8. **Meanwhile, make the ganache:** Place the chopped chocolate in a heatproof bowl. In a small saucepan, bring the cream to a strong simmer over medium heat. Pour the hot cream over the chocolate and let sit for 3 minutes to melt the chocolate. Whisk until the mixture is completely smooth and then let stand for 20 minutes to slightly thicken.

9. Invert the cake onto a wire cooling rack set over a sheet tray. Remove the parchment round. Drizzle the ganache over the top of the cooled cake and then sprinkle the remaining pecans around the perimeter of the top. Transfer the cake to a large plate or cake stand, slice, and serve. Store for up to 3 days covered.

Pumpkin Pie

Serves 8

Crust

2½ cups **unbleached, nonbromated flour**

½ teaspoon **ground cinnamon**

½ teaspoon **kosher salt**

12 tablespoons (1½ sticks) **unsalted butter**, cubed and chilled

¼ cup ice **water**

Filling

1 (15-ounce) can **unsweetened pumpkin puree** (not pumpkin pie filling)

1 cup **unsweetened full-fat coconut milk**

3 large **eggs**

½ cup **pure maple syrup**

2 teaspoons **vanilla extract**

2 teaspoons **freshly grated nutmeg**

1 teaspoon **ground cinnamon**

Grated zest of ½ orange

Kosher salt

If I've learned anything from hosting years of Thanksgiving dinners, it's this: Don't mess with the pumpkin pie! So when this version, made with zero granulated sugar, did not start a family feud, I knew it was a keeper. Pumpkin and maple syrup are made for each other, and the orange zest provides a citrusy boost. This might be the most pumpkin-y pumpkin pie you ever taste. Buy a gluten-free pie shell to make this a flour-free pumpkin pie experience.

1. **Make the crust:** In a food processor, pulse together the flour, cinnamon, and salt. Add the butter and pulse until small crumbs form, about 5 times. With the processor running, add the ice water. Stop the processor when the dough begins to come together in a ball. Transfer the dough to a large sheet of plastic wrap and press into a ball so it holds together. Then flatten the dough into a 1-inch-thick disc, wrap in plastic wrap, and refrigerate for at least 2 hours or up to overnight.

2. Remove the dough from the refrigerator and allow it to come to room temperature, about 15 minutes, then unwrap it and set it on a lightly floured surface. Use a rolling pin to roll the dough until it is about 2 inches wider than a 9-inch pie pan. Brush off excess flour from the dough before laying it into the pan and gently fitting it into the bottom and sides of the pan. Trim the edge of the dough so there is a 1-inch overhang. Fold and crimp the edges of the dough and then prick the bottom of the dough about 5 times with a fork and freeze uncovered for 10 minutes or up to overnight if covered.

3. Preheat the oven to 350°F.

▶ Recipe continues

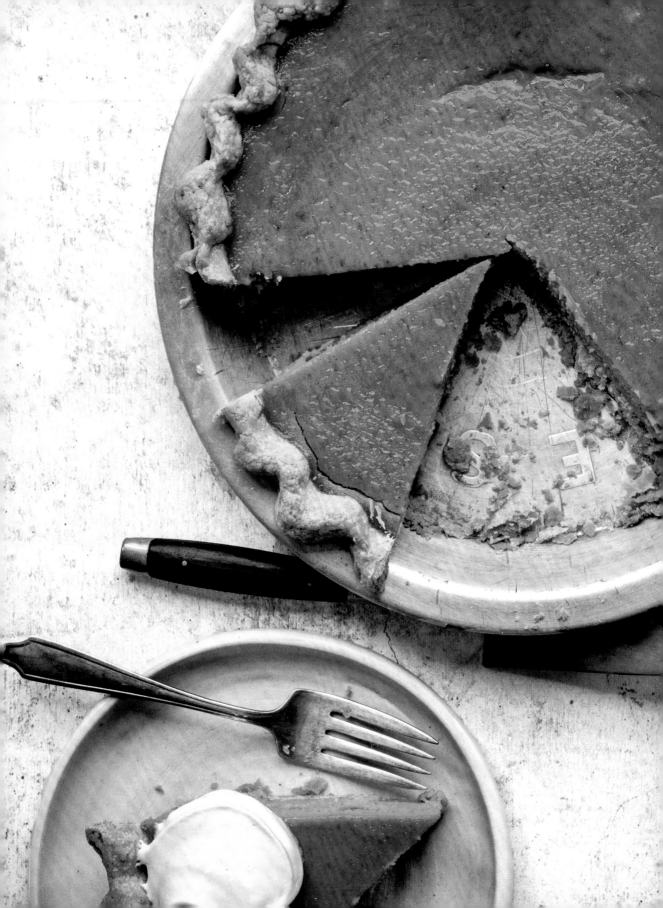

4. Fit a large piece of parchment paper into the pie shell and fill with pie weights or dried beans. Bake until the sides are set, about 30 minutes. Remove the piecrust from the oven, carefully remove the parchment paper and the weights, then return to the oven and continue baking until the crust is light golden brown, about 15 minutes more.

5. **Meanwhile, make the filling:** In a large bowl, whisk together the pumpkin, coconut milk, eggs, maple syrup, vanilla, nutmeg, cinnamon, orange zest, and a pinch of salt. Pour this mixture into the piecrust and continue baking until the filling is set, about 1 hour 15 minutes.

6. Remove the pie from the oven and cool for at least 1 hour before slicing and serving. Store for up to 3 days covered in the fridge.

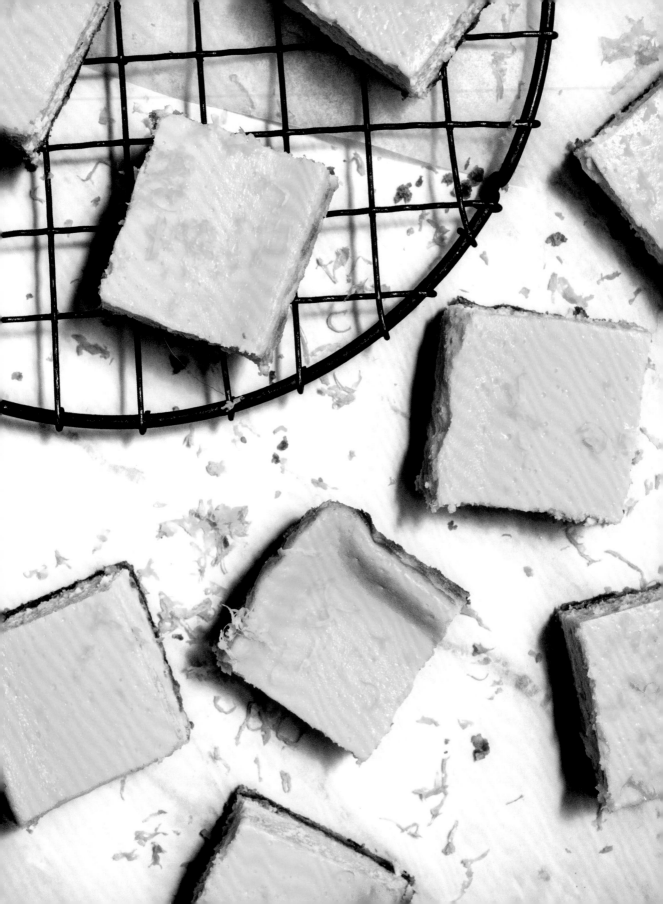

Gluten-Free Lemon Cheesecake Squares

**Makes twenty-four
2-inch squares**

Crust

½ cup raw **cashew pieces**

2 cups **almond flour**

1 teaspoon **ground ginger**

Kosher salt

3 tablespoons **unsalted butter**, melted

1 tablespoon **raw honey**

Filling

3 (8-ounce) bricks **cream cheese**, at room temperature

1 cup **sour cream**

¾ cup **raw honey**

Grated zest of 3 lemons

¼ teaspoon **kosher salt**

5 large **eggs**

1 teaspoon **vanilla extract**

Lemon zest (optional)

If you love cheesecake as much as I do, you'll dig this recipe. This version is as light as air, has a great lemony punch, and sidesteps the typical cup or two of granulated sugar for some honey. The result is a delicate and elegant dessert with a great (gluten-free) crust.

1. Preheat the oven to 350°F.

2. **Make the crust:** In a food processor, pulse the cashews until they become a fine crumb, about 10 times. Add the almond flour, ginger, and a pinch of salt and pulse a couple times to combine. Pour this mixture into a medium bowl, add the melted butter and honey, and stir with a fork to combine until it resembles coarse meal. Press the mixture evenly onto the bottom of a 9 × 13-inch baking pan. Bake until light golden brown, about 15 minutes. Remove from the oven and set aside.

3. Reduce the oven temperature to 300°F.

4. **Make the filling:** In a stand mixer fitted with the paddle, beat together the cream cheese and blend on medium-high speed until completely smooth, about 2 minutes. Mix in the sour cream, honey, lemon zest, and salt on medium speed, occasionally scraping down the sides of the bowl, until the mixture is smooth, about 2 minutes. With the mixer running on low speed, add the eggs one at a time. Add the vanilla and mix to combine.

5. Pour the batter onto the crust. Return to the oven and bake until it begins to brown around the edges and the center is set, about 1 hour. Remove from the oven and allow to cool slightly. While still warm, slice into 24 squares, then cover the pan with plastic wrap and chill until cold. Garnish with lemon zest, if desired, and serve chilled. Store for up to 3 days covered in the fridge.

Drinks and Snacks

Like most people, I don't eat just when I'm hungry; I eat when I'm bored, sad, anxious, stressed out . . . you name it! In the past, I would do what most people did and just reach for a bag of store-bought snacks that are loaded with sugars, stabilizers, salt, and other processed junk that really does a number on my physical well-being. To avoid feeling lousy when hunger (or boredom, or stress . . .) strikes, I make sure that I have fruits and vegetables to make juices and smoothies, as well as the healthy, homemade snacks in this chapter to see me through.

Depending on the ingredients, smoothies can range from wholesome and beneficial health supplements all the way down to delicious but nutritionally barren drinks that better resemble milkshakes. I rely on smoothies for their ability to act as quick and nutritious meal replacements, healthy afternoon pick-me-ups, and tools that help me manage inflammation. Some are a great source of protein, others are loaded with antioxidants and minerals, and most of them (maybe not the green ones) can be handed off to unsuspecting kids as delicious treats.

Instead of a juicer, I like to use a high-powered blender to make smoothies because they work faster and clean easier, and you get the added benefits of fiber, which is especially helpful if you're using a smoothie as a meal replacer. When shopping for smoothies and juices in the real world, remember that they are like anything else. Some are transparently fresh, healthy, and beneficial, while others might be loaded with additives like sugars, preservatives, and stabilizers. Also know that products that undergo heat-pasteurization will lack much of the beneficial bacteria, antioxidants, and nutrients found in freshly made juice. While fresher is always better when it comes to fruit and vegetable smoothies, these will all keep fine overnight in the fridge. Whole milk, cashew milk, almond milk, soy milk, and oat milk are interchangeable in these recipes, so feel free to swap.

Blue Booster,
page 216

Peanut Butter Protein
Shake, page 215

Green Smoothie,
page 227

Peanut Butter Protein Shake

Makes 1 shake (2½ cups)

1 ripe **banana**, peeled

6 large **strawberries**, hulled

3 tablespoons store-bought or homemade **creamy organic peanut butter** (page 249)

1 cup **milk** (your choice)

1 cup **ice**

½ teaspoon **ground cinnamon**

The only way to improve on a peanut butter and banana smoothie is by adding sweet strawberries and turning it into the smoothie version of PB&J! This is my go-to shake after my morning workout, when my body is craving protein. It is getting a lot easier to find markets and grocery stores that make and sell freshly ground peanut butter. I urge you to look for one because it really makes a big difference in terms of flavor and freshness, not to mention the fact that most commercial brands add sugar and hydrogenated oils to keep the spread from separating. Me, I'd rather stir than ingest trans fats. Better still, make your own peanut butter using the recipe on page 249. If you are trying to avoid dairy, you can swap the milk out for almond or oat milk.

In a high-powered blender, add the ingredients in the order listed. Process until smooth.

Blue Booster

**Makes 1 smoothie
(2½ cups)**

1 cup **spinach leaves**

1 cup chopped **kale leaves**, tough stems removed

1 cup **blueberries**

1 teaspoon grated **fresh ginger**

1 teaspoon grated **fresh turmeric** or ½ teaspoon **ground turmeric**

Juice of ½ lemon

½ teaspoon **freshly ground black pepper**

1 cup **water**

1 cup **ice**

This might not be the prettiest drink in the world, but it is the best in terms of helping my body recover from cheat meals and lapses in judgment, if you know what I mean. It's loaded with spinach, kale, and blueberries, superfoods that get me back on track fast. Don't skimp on the freshly ground black pepper; it's not in there for heat, but to help your body better absorb the beneficial curcumin in the turmeric.

In a high-powered blender, add the ingredients in the order listed. Process until smooth.

Apple Beet Ginger Carrot Juice

Makes 1 serving (2½ cups)

½ **Granny Smith apple**, unpeeled, cored, and roughly chopped

1 small **red beet**, peeled and roughly chopped

1 medium organic **carrot**, unpeeled and roughly chopped

1 tablespoon grated **fresh ginger**

1½ cups **water**

Juice of 1 medium orange

Ginger has long been used for its amazing medicinal properties. It's great for treating nausea, aiding digestion, and even helping to fight off colds and flus, but I love it for its powerful anti-inflammatory qualities. When I'm looking for a quick, easy, and delicious way to pack more fruits and raw veggies into my day, this refreshing smoothie definitely does the trick.

In a blender, combine all the ingredients and process until smooth. Serve over ice.

Banana-Lime Smoothie

Makes 1 smoothie (2½ cups)

2 ripe **bananas**, peeled

Grated zest and juice of ½ lime

1 tablespoon **raw honey**

1 cup **Turmeric Milk** (page 245)

1 teaspoon **Oregano Oil** (page 244)

This smoothie is delicious medicine in a glass. It's filling and satisfying and loaded with health-enhancing foods like oregano and turmeric. Those same compounds responsible for oregano's distinctive aroma, called phenols, have remarkable antibacterial qualities, and turmeric is tops at countering inflammation. Again, if you are trying to avoid dairy, you can swap the milk out for almond or oat milk.

In a blender, combine all the ingredients and process until smooth.

Spiced Walnuts

Makes 2½ cups

2 tablespoons **extra-virgin olive oil**

2 cups **walnut halves**

¼ cup **raw honey**

1 tablespoon finely chopped **fresh rosemary**

1 teaspoon **ground ginger**

½ teaspoon **kosher salt**

¼ teaspoon **ground cinnamon**

¼ teaspoon **cayenne pepper**

I try to come up with different ways to use walnuts because they are always available, are way less expensive than other nuts, and are chock-full of antioxidants. They also have more omega-3 fatty acids than any other nut, and omega-3s are proven to fight inflammation and joint pain. I like to have these around during the holidays when people are always dropping by and reaching for a salty snack.

1. Line a sheet pan with parchment paper.

2. Set a large heavy-bottomed skillet over medium heat. Add the olive oil and heat to shimmering, then add the walnuts. Cook, stirring occasionally, until lightly toasted, about 3 minutes. Add the honey, rosemary, ginger, salt, cinnamon, and cayenne and cook, stirring occasionally, until the walnuts are golden brown and fragrant, about 2 minutes.

3. Arrange the nuts in a single layer on the prepared sheet pan and set aside to cool, about 20 minutes. Once cool, break up any large clumps with your hands. Store in an airtight container for up to 3 days.

Drinks and Snacks

Spring Pea Hummus

Serves 4

Kosher salt and freshly ground black pepper

2 cups **fresh peas**

¼ cup roughly chopped **ramps**, leaves and bulbs, or scallions

½ cup roughly chopped **fresh flat-leaf parsley**

¼ cup **fresh lemon juice**, plus more as neeeded

3 tablespoons **tahini**

¾ cup **extra-virgin olive oil**, plus more for bread

1 **baguette**, cut into ¾-inch-thick slices

Each spring at Lola, my restaurant in Cleveland, we peel bushels of garden peas before service. I'm not talking about removing the peas from their tough outer jackets; I mean separating the delicate meat from its paper-thin coating. Each pea, one by one, by hand. Don't worry, you don't have to do that for this recipe because we blend it all up. I think of English peas as nature's candy, and they make an amazingly light and fresh version of hummus. If you can't score some wild ramps (available in the spring) at a farmers' market, go ahead and substitute scallions. This bright and springy spread works great on slices of toasted baguette, but if you're avoiding flour, you can also serve it under or alongside Yogurt-Roasted Chicken (page 142) or Slow-Roasted Salmon (page 87).

1. Set up an ice bath by filling a medium bowl with ice and water. In a medium saucepan, bring 8 cups water and 1 tablespoon salt to a boil over high heat. Add the peas and cook until just tender, about 1 minute. Drain and then plunge them into the ice bath to cool. Drain again and transfer to a kitchen towel to dry.

2. In a blender or food processer, combine the peas, ramps, parsley, lemon juice, tahini, and a big pinch of salt. Process until smooth. With the machine running, slowly add the ¾ cup olive oil in a steady stream. Taste and adjust for seasoning, adding salt and/or lemon as needed. Scrape into a bowl, cover with plastic wrap and refrigerate until serving (or up to 3 days).

3. Preheat a grill or grill pan to medium-high heat.

4. Brush both sides of the baguette slices with olive oil, season with salt and pepper, and place on the grill. Cook until slightly charred and toasted on both sides, about 1 minute per side. Serve the hummus with the grilled bread on the side.

Overnight Chia Seed Pudding
with Fresh Berries and Bee Pollen

Serves 4

Chia seeds are tiny nutritional powerhouses that are loaded with antioxidants, omega-3 fatty acids, protein, and more. The beauty of this recipe is that all the work happens overnight in the fridge while you're sound asleep. After sitting all night, the seeds plump up and get this soft, silky texture that reminds me of the rice pudding I ate as a kid. Top this with whatever ripe seasonal fruit is on hand and, if you have it, bee pollen, which boosts immunity, fights inflammation, and adds a nice little crunch.

2 cups **unsweetened full-fat coconut milk**

2 tablespoons **pure maple syrup** or **raw honey**, plus more as neeeded

⅛ teaspoon **ground cinnamon**

1 teaspoon **vanilla extract**

Kosher salt

¼ cup **chia seeds**

¼ cup **unsweetened shredded coconut**

1 cup **blackberries**

1 cup pitted **cherries**, halved

¼ cup **bee pollen**

1. In a large bowl, whisk together the coconut milk, maple syrup, cinnamon, vanilla, and a pinch of salt. Taste and adjust for sweetness, adding more maple syrup as needed. Add the chia seeds and coconut and stir well to combine. Cover the bowl with plastic wrap and refrigerate overnight.

2. To serve, spoon the mixture into bowls and top with fresh blackberries, cherries, and bee pollen.

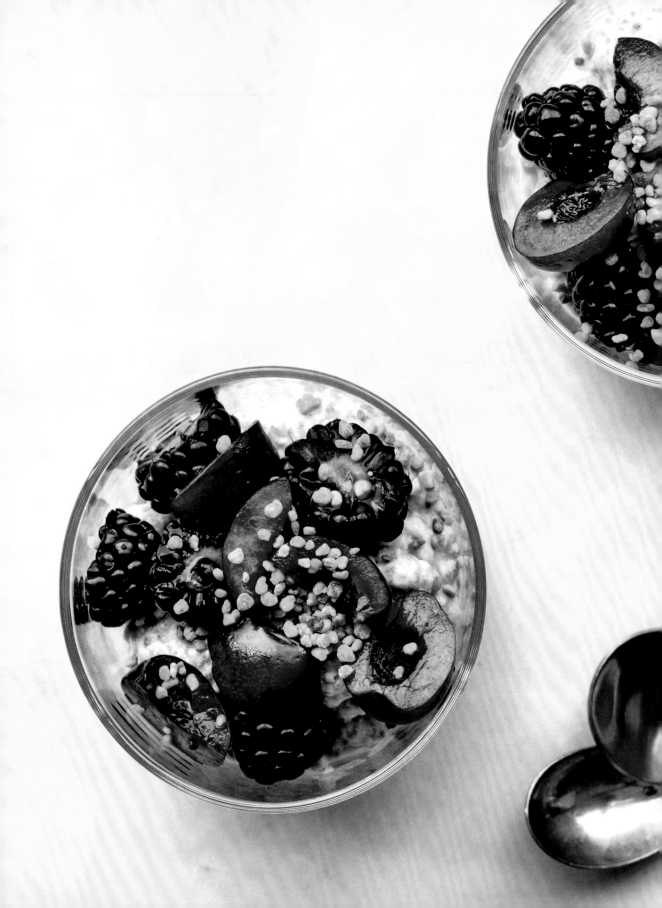

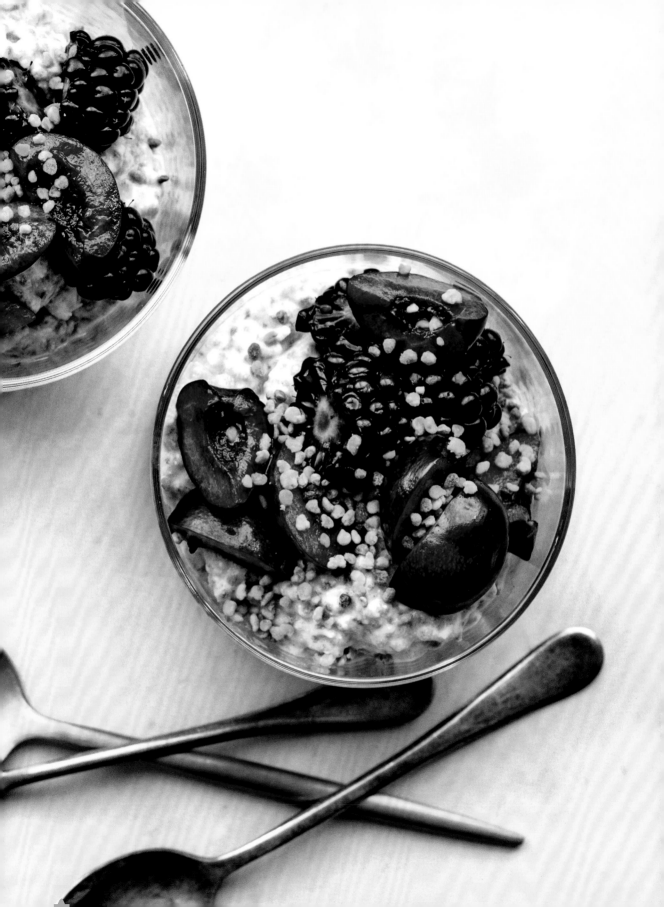

Pineapple, Blackberry, and Basil Smoothie

Makes 1 smoothie (2½ cups)

1 cup chopped **fresh pineapple**

1 cup **blackberries**

½ cup **basil leaves**

1 cup **coconut water**

Juice of ½ lime

One sip of this great smoothie and you'll swear you're hanging out on some tropical island. This bright and festive drink goes down great on a hot summer day when you're lounging outside or working in the garden. The coconut water brings vitamins and minerals to the party that regular water does not. And if you're feeling a little rowdy, you can add a shot of rum to turn it into a tasty cocktail. After all, life is all about balance!

In a blender, combine all the ingredients and process until smooth.

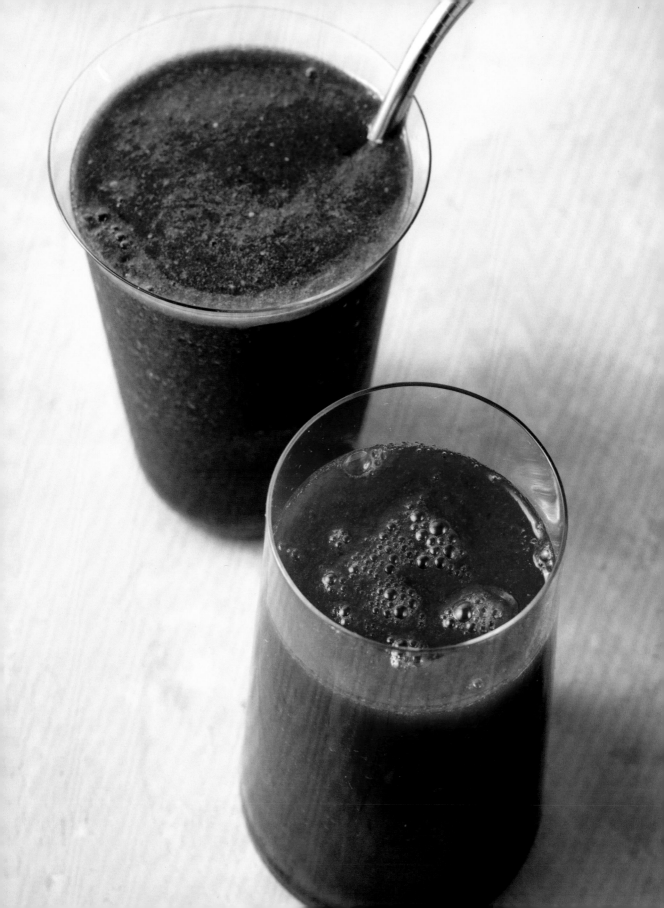

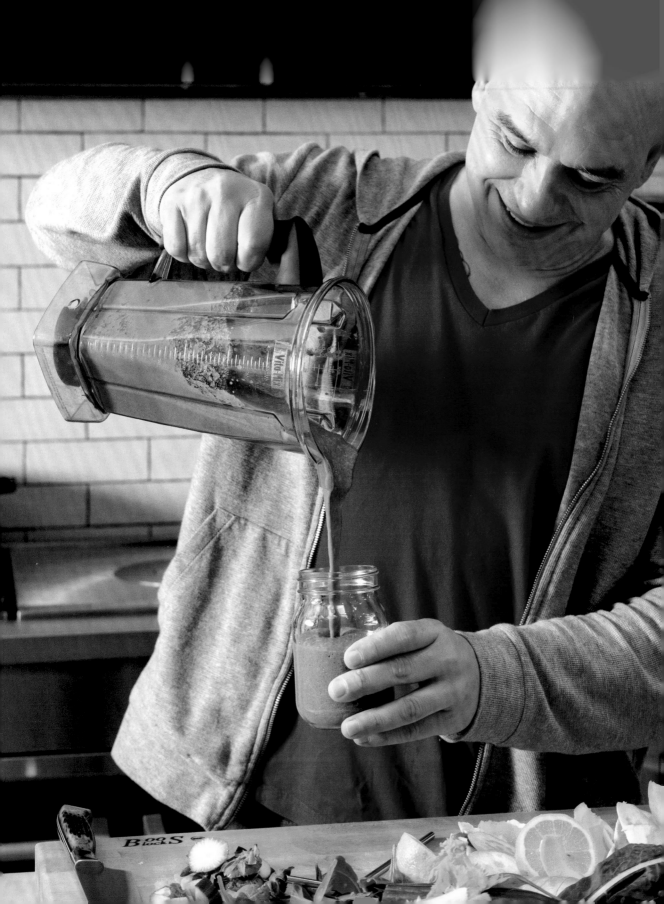

Green Smoothie

**Makes 1 smoothie
(2½ cups)**

1 cup **spinach leaves**

1 cup chopped **kale leaves**, tough stems removed

½ cup **seedless green grapes**

½ **Granny Smith apple**, unpeeled and roughly chopped

1 tablespoon grated **fresh ginger**

1 cup **water**

1 cup **ice**

Green juices have gotten a bad rap because so many of them are just plain awful—awful to look at and to drink. Not this version, which will make a convert out of anyone, as it did me! This one combines the natural sweetness of grapes and apple with the superfood benefits of spinach, kale, and ginger. Not only is it full of fiber, it tastes amazing and costs almost nothing compared to those fancy juice-shop bottles.

In a blender, combine all the ingredients and process until smooth.

Ginger-Lemon-Verbena Tea

Makes 1 to 2 cups

¼ cup **fresh ginger juice** (see note)

Juice of ½ lemon

3 **whole cloves**

¼ teaspoon **Cayenne Oil** (page 246)

15 **fresh lemon verbena leaves**
  or 3 tablespoons dried leaves

Honey (optional)

Note For the ginger juice, you can buy some from a juice bar, juice it yourself at home, or grate ginger on a micro-plane/rasp-style grater and add the juicy pulp to a sieve, then press on it to extract the juice.

Sometimes you need a hot, steaming mug of something comforting and soothing. Beef Bone Broth (page 237) works great for that, and so does this tea, which I drink on days when I'm feeling a little under the weather and want something light and simple, yet warming to drink. Not only is ginger a great anti-inflammatory, it works miracles on upset stomachs and nausea. I sometimes swap out my late-afternoon coffee for a cup of this and don't even miss it. You can usually find fresh lemon verbena where other herbs are sold, but dried leaves will work, too.

1. In a medium saucepan, combine 1½ cups water, the ginger juice, lemon juice, cloves, Cayenne Oil, and lemon verbena. Bring to a simmer over medium heat. Turn off the heat, cover the pan, and steep for 5 minutes.

2. Strain the tea into a mug and serve. If you like a touch of sweetness, add a squirt of honey.

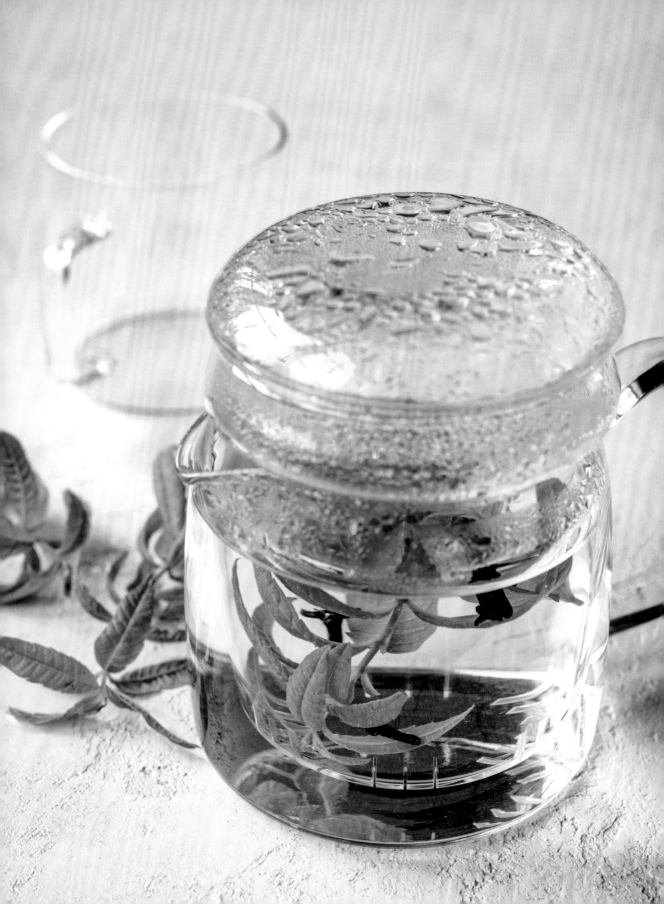

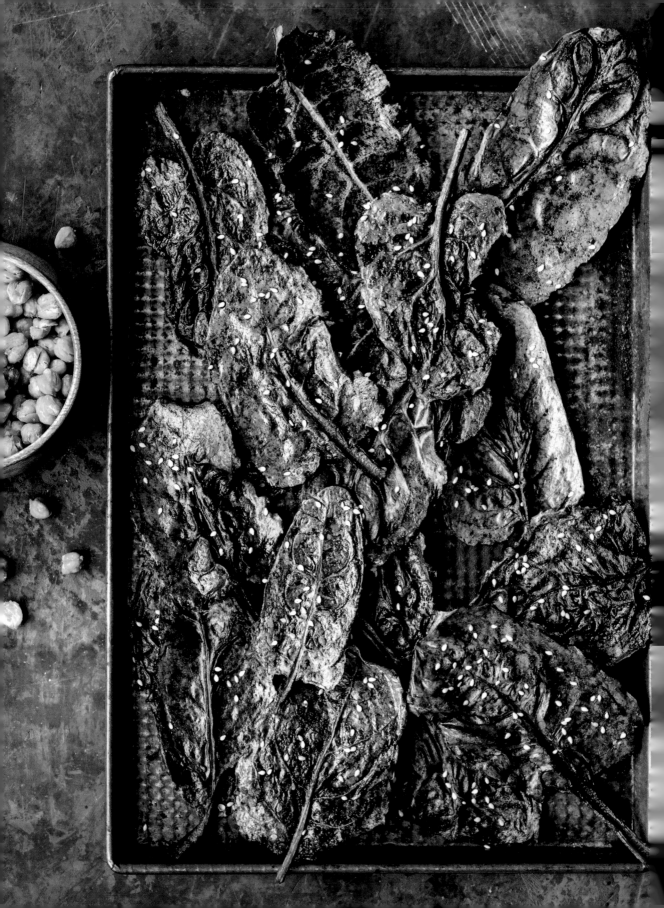

Chili and Garlic Swiss Chard Chips

Serves 2 to 4

2 tablespoons **extra-virgin olive oil**

1 teaspoon **chili powder**

½ teaspoon **garlic powder**

¼ teaspoon **kosher salt**

½ pound **Swiss chard**, stems removed and leaves sliced into 3-inch squares

1 tablespoon **white sesame seeds**

Like most people, I love baked kale chips. But not all kale chips are made equal. Some are too cheesy, others are too salty, and still others have an unpleasant bitter aftertaste. On my quest to make a better kale chip, I ended up ditching the kale altogether and going with Swiss chard leaves! These crispy snacks are loaded with antioxidants and vitamins C and K, and are a good source of iron. They get a nice little kick from the chili powder and added crunch from the nutty sesame seeds.

1. Preheat the oven to 300°F. Line 2 sheet pans with parchment paper.

2. In a large bowl, whisk to combine the olive oil, chili powder, garlic powder, and salt. Add the Swiss chard and toss to coat so both sides of the leaves are well seasoned.

3. Arrange the Swiss chard in a single layer on the prepared sheet pans, making sure to leave some space between the leaves. Sprinkle with the sesame seeds and bake until the leaves begin to brown and crisp, about 10 minutes. Flip the leaves and continue cooking until they are completely crisp, about 10 minutes more.

4. Serve immediately or store in an airtight container for up to 1 day.

Crispy Baked Chickpeas

Makes 1 cup

1 (15-ounce) can **chickpeas**, drained and rinsed

1 tablespoon **extra-virgin olive oil**

½ teaspoon **kosher salt**

These salty, crunchy little snacks are completely addicting and a great source of meat-free protein. I make double (or triple) batches and eat them straight out of the jar. But I also use them as flour-free toppings for salads, soups, and seafood dishes when I want to add a little texture. I know that peeling chickpeas sounds insane, but it makes a huge difference in terms of crispiness, both immediately and for a few days after you make them. Just pop them out of their skins with your thumb and forefinger. Pretend it's your moment of Zen!

1. Preheat the oven to 350°F.

2. Spread the chickpeas out on a dry kitchen towel, top with a second towel, and gently press and roll them around with your hands to loosen the skins. Use your fingers to remove any that haven't fallen off. (Discard the skins.)

3. In a medium bowl, toss together the chickpeas, olive oil, and salt.

4. Arrange the chickpeas in a single layer on a sheet pan and cook, occasionally shaking the pan, until the chickpeas are crispy and golden brown, about 40 minutes.

5. Remove the sheet pan from the oven. If you'd like to season with your favorite spices, do that now. Allow them to cool completely before storing in an airtight container for up to 3 days in the pantry.

Strawberry Fruit Roll-Ups

Makes 8 roll-ups

1 pound **strawberries**, hulled

¼ cup **raw honey**

Kosher salt

2 tablespoons **fresh lemon juice**

I used to love snacking on packaged fruit roll-ups when I was a kid. What I didn't know (or care about) back then was the fact that they are made with corn syrup, food colorings, and other weird and totally artificial ingredients. This recipe is just real fruit and honey—and you can literally smell and taste the difference. Roll-ups are a great way to utilize ripe, in-season fruit because the roll-up will last for a month in your pantry and up to a year in the freezer. They might take a long time to cook, but it's largely hands-off time, and the results speak for themselves.

1. Preheat the oven to 180°F. Line a sheet pan with a silicone baking mat.

2. In a blender or food processer, process the strawberries until completely smooth, about 30 seconds. Strain through a fine-mesh sieve set over a medium bowl to remove most of the seeds (it's okay if some remain). Add the honey and a pinch of salt to the strawberries and whisk to combine.

3. Transfer the strawberry mixture to a nonreactive medium saucepan and cook over medium heat, stirring occasionally, until it has a thick, jam-like consistency, about 15 minutes. Remove from the heat and stir in the lemon juice.

4. Spread the strawberry mixture in a thin, even layer on the silicone-lined sheet pan. Bake until the surface is no longer tacky, about 4 hours. Remove from the oven and allow to cool for 1 hour.

5. Cut a piece of wax paper to the size and shape of the sheet pan and lay it on top of the cooled fruit leather, lightly pressing to affix. Invert the fruit leather so the wax paper is on the bottom. Carefully remove the silicone and then cut the fruit-lined wax paper lengthwise into 8 long strips. Roll the wax paper and store the fruit roll-ups in an airtight container for up to 1 week.

Strawberry Fruit
Roll-Ups, page 233

Coconut-Cashew Granola

Makes 10 cups

4 cups **old-fashioned rolled oats**

2 cups **unsweetened shredded or flaked coconut**

2 cups **slivered almonds**

1 cup **whole raw cashews**

2 teaspoons **ground cinnamon**

1 teaspoon **kosher salt**

¾ cup **extra-virgin olive oil**

½ cup **raw honey**

2 cups **dried fruit**, such as pitted dates, cherries, and/or apricots, roughly chopped

For as long as I've known Liz, she has been making her own granola. It's easy, delicious, and so much more economical than the stuff you buy in stores. Making it at home also puts you in control of the ingredients. For example, instead of using refined sugar or corn syrup as a sweetener, I use raw local honey. This version is loaded with fiber and protein from the almonds and cashews. You might think it's odd to call for so much oil—and olive oil at that—but it creates the perfect toasted finish while adding a surprising amount of flavor. As the granola cools, it will get crispier and crispier.

1. Preheat the oven to 325°F. Line a sheet pan with parchment paper.

2. In a large bowl, toss together the oats, coconut, almonds, cashews, cinnamon, salt, olive oil, and honey.

3. Arrange the mixture in a single layer on the prepared sheet pan and cook, stirring halfway through baking, until golden brown and toasted, about 30 minutes. Allow the granola to cool completely before stirring in the dried fruit. Store in an airtight container for up to 1 week.

Pantry Staples

To help me manage my inflammation and discomfort through food, cooking, and diet, I've come to rely on a small stable of essential pantry items. Things like homemade bone broth, sauerkraut, Dairy-Free Parmesan, Turmeric Milk, Cayenne Oil, and others have come to the rescue so many times in my daily cooking that I try to never be without. I know that making some of these recipes might seem like a lot of work, but I think that you'll discover not only that the results are more than worth it, but also that they are pretty fun projects to undertake. Not only that, most of these items store for weeks or even months, so you only need to make them a couple times a year.

Beef Bone Broth

Makes 4 quarts

6 to 7 pounds **beef bones** (shin, knuckle, neck, marrow, oxtail; ask your butcher to cut them into pieces that will fit in your stockpot)

1 tablespoon **extra-virgin olive oil**

¼ cup **raw unfiltered apple cider vinegar with mother**

2 **yellow onions**, halved

4 medium **carrots**, cut into 1-inch pieces

1 head **garlic**, loose papery skin removed, halved through the equator

1 bunch **flat-leaf parsley**

1 small bundle **fresh thyme**

3 **bay leaves**, dried or fresh

2 tablespoons **kosher salt**

1 tablespoon **black peppercorns**

For serving

Grated **fresh turmeric** or **ground turmeric**

Grated **fresh ginger**

Lemon wedges

Freshly ground black pepper

I was first exposed to the miracles of bone broth by my friend Marco Canora, the chef and owner of Hearth restaurant in New York. He deserves credit for kick-starting the whole modern bone-broth craze. While this supercharged version of beef stock has been around for ages, Canora helped shine fresh light on its amazing qualities. After incorporating bone broth into his daily routine and experiencing firsthand its numerous health benefits, Canora launched Brodo, a quick-serve business built around steaming mugs of bone broth. I was skeptical at first about all the claims swirling around this now-trendy food, but I couldn't argue with the results. Since making them a regular part of my routine, bone broths have helped me in countless ways, from lifting my mood and easing joint pain, to reducing hunger and settling my stomach. The vinegar in this recipe is one of the elements that separates beef stock from bone broth as it—along with the really long cook times—helps to extract components like collagen, minerals, and amino acids from the sturdy beef bones. It really is as close to a perfectly balanced and nutritious food as I can imagine. I prefer to use organic vegetables and bones from grass-fed beef. If you have any mushrooms, or even mushroom stems, go ahead and toss them into the pot for added health benefits. The selenium in them is a strong antioxidant.

1. Preheat the oven to 450°F. Line a sheet pan with foil.

2. Arrange the beef bones in a single layer on the sheet pan. Lightly drizzle with the olive oil and roast until golden brown, about 45 minutes.

▶ Recipe continues

3. Transfer the bones to a large stockpot and add cold water to cover by 2 to 3 inches. Add the vinegar and bring to a gentle boil over high heat. Reduce the heat to low and simmer the stock uncovered for 1 hour, occasionally skimming off the scummy foam that rises to the surface with a fine-mesh sieve or ladle.

4. Add the onions, carrots, garlic, parsley, thyme, bay leaves, salt, and peppercorns and continue cooking over low heat, uncovered, for 12 hours, occasionally skimming off any excess fat or scummy foam that rises to the surface.

5. Use tongs to remove and discard the bones. Strain the broth through a fine-mesh sieve and into a 4-quart heatproof container or several smaller containers. Discard the solids.

6. To serve, ladle the broth into cups or bowls and garnish with turmeric and ginger. Add a squeeze of lemon and some freshly cracked pepper to taste. To store, refrigerate in airtight containers for up to 5 days or up to 1 month in the freezer.

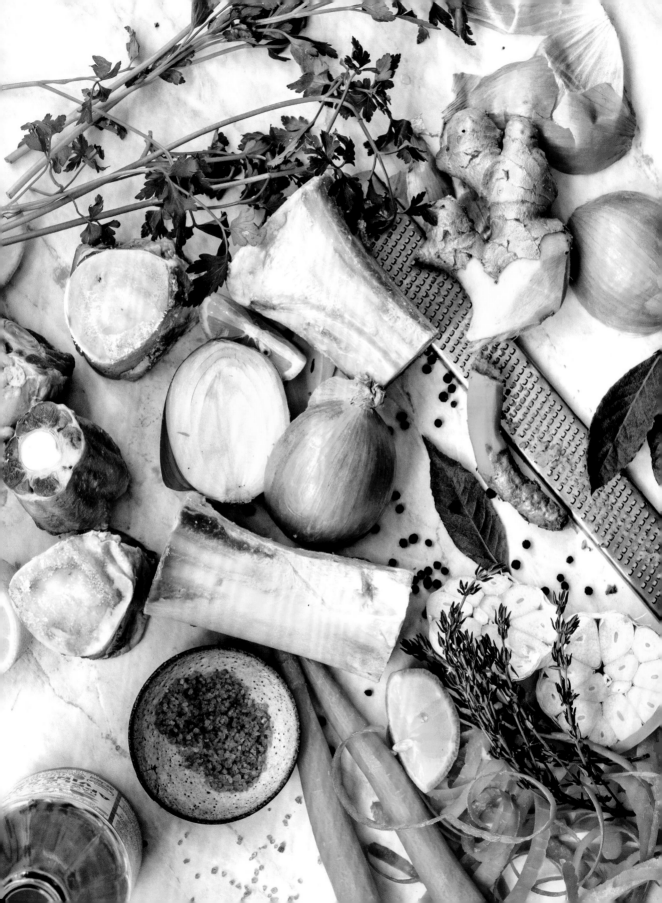

Vegetable Stock

Makes 3 quarts

3 **leeks**, white and light-green parts, cut crosswise into 3-inch lengths

1 **fennel bulb**, cored and quartered

4 **celery ribs**, cut crosswise into 3-inch lengths

1 head **garlic**, halved through the equator

3 medium **carrots**, unpeeled and cut crosswise into 3-inch lengths

1 tablespoon **coriander seeds**

1 teaspoon **black peppercorns**

2 **fresh bay leaves**

Small bundle **fresh parsley**

Small bundle **fresh thyme**

1 cup **mushrooms stems** or 2 cups whole button mushrooms

Pinch of **kosher salt**

There's almost nothing easier than making a big pot of vegetable stock, and its uses are almost limitless. It makes the perfect jumping-off point for a million different soups, you can add it to stews and braises, or use it to get just the right consistency in sauces. I also like to substitute it in place of water when cooking rice, polenta, and couscous for a richer flavor.

In a large stockpot, combine all of the ingredients and cover with 1 gallon (16 cups) cold water. Bring the water to a strong simmer over medium-high heat. Reduce the heat to medium-low and cook, partially covered, until the vegetables begin sinking, about 1½ hours. Strain into several airtight containers, chill, and refrigerate for up to 3 days or freeze up to 1 month.

Mushroom Stock

Makes 3 quarts (12 cups)

½ bunch **fresh thyme**

2 ounces **dried shiitake or porcini mushrooms** (about ¼ cup)

4 cups roughly chopped **fresh button or cremini mushrooms**

1 **yellow onion**, roughly chopped

3 medium **carrots**, unpeeled and roughly chopped

2 **celery ribs**, roughly chopped

2 **fresh bay leaves**

1 tablespoon **black peppercorns**

2 tablespoons **kosher salt**

According to the people who follow these sorts of things, mushroom stock is having a "moment." I'm not sure what that means, but I do know that it is one of the easiest and most economical stocks to make at home, and the resulting elixir adds incredible depth and richness to all manner of soups, stews, and grain dishes. We call for it in Wild Mushroom Risotto (page 55) and Couscous with Lentils, Kimchi, Peas, and Mushrooms (page 183), where the brew imparts extra earthiness.

In a large stockpot, combine all of the ingredients and cover with 1 gallon (16 cups) cold water. Bring to a gentle boil over medium-high heat. Reduce to low and simmer, partially covered, for 1½ hours. Strain, chill, and store for up to 3 days in the fridge and up to 1 month in the freezer.

Dairy-Free Parmesan

Makes 1¼ cups

1 cup **raw cashews**

¼ cup **nutritional yeast**

½ teaspoon **garlic powder**

¾ teaspoon **kosher salt**

I'm not going to claim that this stuff tastes exactly like real Parmigiano-Reggiano, because there's only one thing in the world that tastes like it, and that's real Parmigiano-Reggiano! But if you have to avoid dairy in your diet and you still want to add a nutty, savory, salty, and "cheesy" flavor to foods, this nut-based vegan alternative is amazing. It is so easy to make that I always have a double or triple recipe stashed in my fridge, where it will last for weeks.

In a blender or food processor, pulse the cashews, nutritional yeast, garlic powder, and salt until the mixture has the consistency of fine crumbs and resembles freshly grated parmesan cheese, about 10 times. Refrigerate in an airtight container for up to 3 weeks.

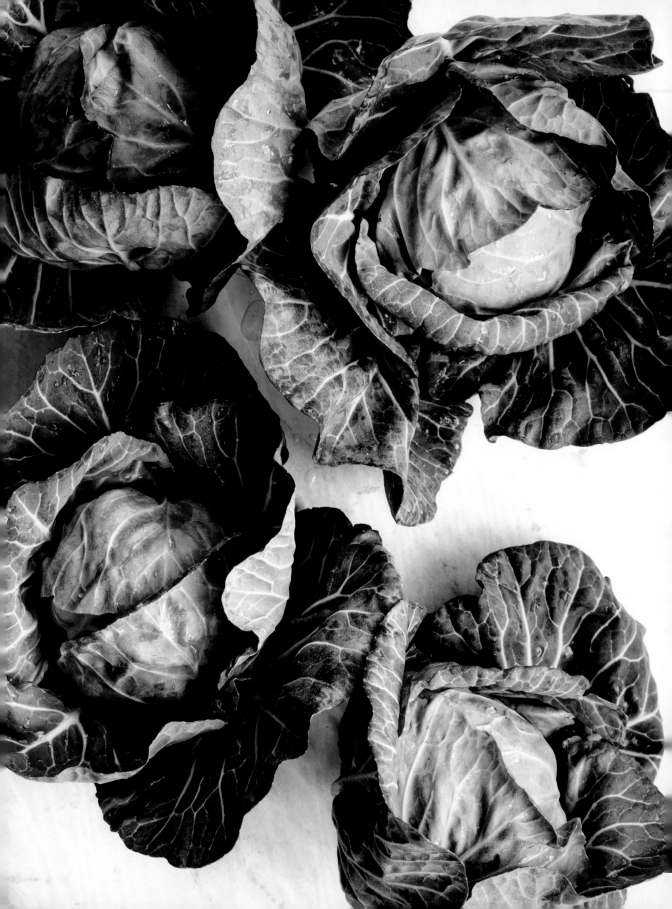

Simple Sauerkraut

Makes 2 quarts

5 pounds **green cabbage**
(about 2 medium heads),
quartered and cored

4 tablespoons **kosher salt**

1 tablespoon **caraway seeds**

I've said it before and I'll say it again: Sauerkraut is a magical food! It is amazing on its own, but it also improves every single food it touches, from bratwurst to burgers. It provides that crucial crunch and twang to succulent braises and slow-roasted meats, and it even goes great on pizza. But best of all are the health benefits of the probiotics, aka beneficial bacteria, that arise from the natural fermentation process. If you suffer from occasional gut issues, probiotics are a great place to start. Sauerkraut is really easy to make—and the longer it ferments, the stronger it gets. Just taste it along the way (it's safe!) and pop it in the fridge when it gets to your liking.

1. Slice each cabbage quarter crosswise into ⅛-inch-wide strips. To rinse, submerge the shredded cabbage in a large container of cold water, then drain in a colander.

2. In a very large bowl, combine the cabbage and salt. With your hands, toss and gently massage the cabbage until it begins to wilt, about 3 minutes. Add the caraway and mix to combine. Set aside until a fair amount of liquid accumulates in the bottom of the bowl, about 15 minutes.

3. Divide the cabbage into two quart-size mason jars, tightly packing the leaves and leaving 2 inches of air space at the top. Divide the liquid evenly between the jars. Place a water-filled drinking glass on top of the cabbage to keep it submerged below the surface of the liquid. Let the jars sit at room temperature to ferment for 7 to 10 days, until the preferred flavor and texture are achieved. Every few days, press down the glass to keep the cabbage submerged below the surface of the liquid.

Oregano Oil

Makes ¾ cup

¾ cup **grapeseed oil**
12 sprigs **fresh oregano**

The very same compounds responsible for oregano's distinctive and delicious smell also happen to possess powerful antibacterial, antifungal, and anti-inflammatory properties. When consumed in recipes like Rolled Spinach Omelet (page 18) and Quinoa and Egg Salad with Chickpeas and Asparagus (page 27), or in beverages like Banana-Lime Smoothie (page 218), I find that oregano oil aids digestion. I also use it externally, rubbing it into stiff and sore joints and muscles for almost immediate relief.

1. In a medium saucepan, combine the grapeseed oil and oregano and cook over low heat until the temperature of the oil reaches 200°F on a digital thermometer, about 2 minutes.

2. Remove the pan from the heat and set aside to cool for 1 hour.

3. Pour the oil through a fine-mesh sieve and into a mason jar, pressing on the oregano to extract as much oil as possible. Refrigerate for up to 2 months.

Quinoa

Makes 3 cups

1 cup **quinoa**, rinsed
Kosher salt

In a medium saucepan, combine 1¾ cups water, the quinoa, and a good pinch of salt. Bring to a boil over medium-high heat, stir, cover, reduce to a simmer, and cook until the quinoa pops open (which releases the circular white germ of the seed) and all the liquid has been absorbed, about 15 minutes. Fluff quinoa before serving.

Batch It It's always a good idea to have some cooked quinoa on hand to give you a head start in the kitchen. It stores well in the fridge, so go ahead and double the recipe. Simply combine 3½ cups of water with 2 cups of quinoa and a good pinch of salt and follow the instructions above to make a 6-cup batch. Refrigerate the quinoa in an airtight container for up to 3 days or freeze in portions that you want and pull as needed.

Turmeric Milk

Makes 2 cups

2 cups **whole milk** (nondairy milk works, too)

2 teaspoons **ground turmeric**

½ teaspoon **freshly ground black pepper**

1 tablespoon **raw honey**

Turmeric has helped me immensely when it comes to managing inflammation due to my arthritis. It takes a little while for the benefits to really show up, so give it a few days or even weeks, and don't get discouraged. I take capsules in the morning, but I also use this recipe for turmeric milk to bump up my intake. It adds an exotic kick to smoothies, coffee, or tea. You can even use it to add some richness to a nice soup, stew, or braise.

1. In a medium saucepan, combine the milk, turmeric, black pepper, and honey and bring to a gentle boil over low heat.

2. Remove the pan from the heat, cover, and let steep for 30 minutes.

3. Pour through a fine-mesh sieve and into an airtight container. Serve immediately or refrigerate for up to 5 days.

Oat Milk

Makes 5 cups

1 cup **old-fashioned rolled oats**

Pinch of salt (optional)

1 tablespoon **raw honey** or **pure maple syrup** (optional)

Oat milk provides a delicious new option in the hunt for nondairy milk substitutes. Not only is it subtly sweet, rich, and satisfying, it's easy, quick, and economical to make at home. These are just some of the reasons why oat milk is quickly outpacing soy milk and almond milk in popularity.

1. In a medium bowl, combine the oats and 4 cups cold water and stir to combine. Allow to soak at room temperature for 1 hour.

2. Drain the oats (discarding the water) and rinse them. Transfer the oats to a blender, add 4 cups fresh water, and the salt and/or sweetener, if using. Blend until completely smooth, about 2 minutes. Strain through a fine-mesh sieve and chill. Keeps up to 5 days in the refrigerator. Shake before using.

Pantry Staples

Cayenne
Oil

Makes ¾ cup

¾ cup **grapeseed oil**

2 fresh **cayenne peppers**, thinly
sliced with seeds and ribs

1 **garlic clove**, sliced

Cayenne oil packs a punch and brings the heat thanks to capsaicin, the active ingredient in chili peppers. In addition to bringing the heat, capsaicin is a powerful topical pain reliever that you can rub into sore muscles and joints as is, or when combined with beeswax to make a salve. Added to foods like Roasted Broccoli with Cauliflower Puree (page 22) or beverages such as Ginger-Lemon-Verbena Tea (page 228), cayenne oil not only adds a nice flavor boost, but also helps to boost a body's immune system.

1. In a medium saucepan, combine the oil, cayenne peppers, and garlic and cook over low heat until the temperature reaches 200°F on a digital thermometer, about 2 minutes.

2. Remove the pan from the heat and set aside to cool, about 1 hour.

3. Pour the oil through a fine-mesh sieve and into an airtight container and refrigerate for up to 2 months.

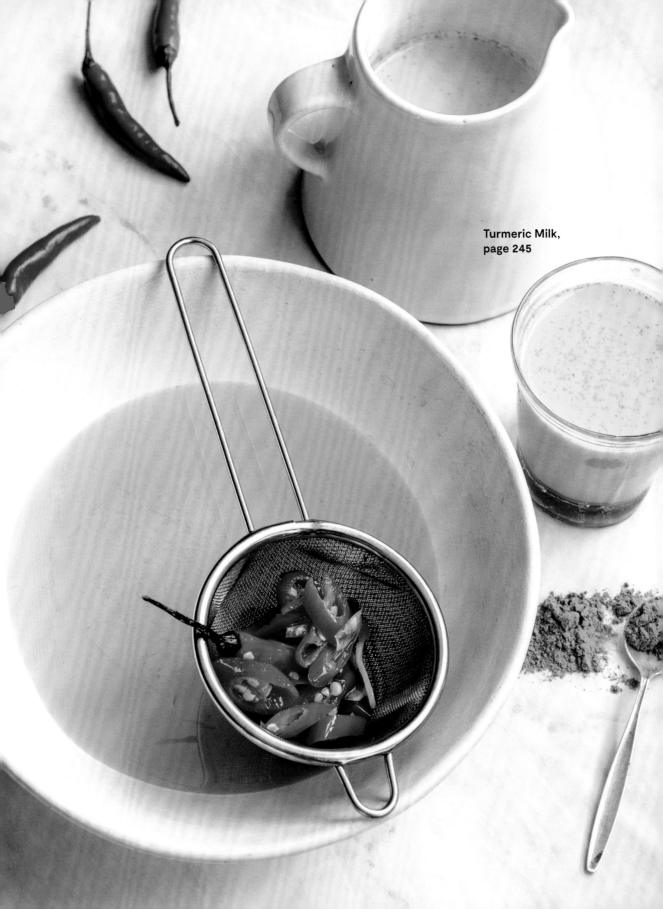

Turmeric Milk,
page 245

Curry Paste

Makes ½ cup

2 tablespoons **coriander seeds**

1 tablespoon **cumin seeds**

1 teaspoon **black peppercorns**

1 teaspoon **fennel seeds**

2 tablespoons **tomato paste**

4 **garlic cloves**, grated on a rasp-style grater

1 tablespoon grated **fresh ginger**

2 teaspoons **ground turmeric**

1 teaspoon **smoked paprika**

½ teaspoon **cayenne pepper**

½ teaspoon **ground cinnamon**

1 teaspoon **kosher salt**

I'd love to tell you that curry powder is a comparable substitute for curry paste, but that would be a lie. Fresh ingredients like garlic and ginger, not to mention the process of freshly toasting and grinding seeds and spices, bring an intensity of aroma and flavor that is impossible to extract from a spice jar. This curry paste, for example, completely transforms dishes like Grilled Mahi Mahi (page 84) and the Chickpea, Kale, and Tomato Stew (page 170). That said, there are some very good jarred curry pastes available at the market if you feel like giving them a try.

1. Place a medium saucepan over medium heat. Add the coriander, cumin, peppercorns, and fennel seeds and toast, stirring occasionally, until warm and fragrant, about 2 minutes. Transfer the spices to a bowl and set aside to cool. Once cool, process the toasted spices to a powder in a spice grinder and set aside.

2. In a medium bowl, mix together the tomato paste, garlic, ginger, turmeric, smoked paprika, cayenne, cinnamon, and salt. Add the ground spice mixture and stir well to combine. Store in an airtight container for up to 3 weeks in the fridge.

Brown Rice

Makes 3 cups

1 cup **brown basmati rice**

Kosher salt

In a medium saucepan, combine 2¼ cups water, the rice, and a good pinch of salt. Bring to a boil over medium-high heat, stir, cover, reduce to a simmer, and cook until the rice is tender and all the liquid has been absorbed, about 45 minutes. Remove from the heat and let stand for 5 minutes.

Batch It Cooked brown rice will last up to 3 days in the fridge. To make a double batch, simply combine 4½ cups of water with 2 cups of brown rice and a good pinch of salt and follow the instructions above to make a 6-cup batch. Cool the rice slightly before refrigerating in an airtight container for up to 3 days.

Homemade Peanut Butter

Makes 1½ cups

2 cups roasted **unsalted peanuts**

2 tablespoons **coconut oil,** melted if solid

¾ teaspoon **vanilla extract**

½ teaspoon **kosher salt**

2 tablespoons **honey** (optional)

So nutty, so creamy, so delicious, so easy. With this recipe, it's important to blend the peanuts while they are still warm from roasting in the oven, which ensures a smooth, velvety texture. Before you reach the desired creamy consistency, the nuts will turn all dry and crumbly; just have faith and keep going. If you want to start with raw, unroasted peanuts, toast them for 5 to 8 minutes at 350°F and then add them straight into the food processor with the rest of the ingredients. This method also works for making other nut and seed butters, like cashew, almond, and sunflower seed.

1. Preheat the oven to 300°F.

2. Arrange the peanuts on a rimmed sheet pan and bake until they begin to appear oily, about 10 minutes.

3. In a food processor fitted with the metal blade, combine the hot peanuts, coconut oil, vanilla, salt, and honey (if using) and blend, occasionally scraping down the sides and bottom of the bowl, until smooth and creamy, about 5 minutes.

4. Scrape the peanut butter into an airtight container and store in the fridge for up to 1 month.

Acknowledgments

Fix It with Food is my sixth cookbook in about ten years, but it's the most personal one I've written to date. In addition to being filled with delicious recipes, the book outlines the process I took to identify the types of foods I can enjoy and those I need to avoid because they trigger inflammation and pain. The experience has helped me immensely—and I hope it will do the same for you. The goal is to be able to still cook and eat amazing foods without ever feeling you're on a diet.

I wouldn't be here without the love and support of Liz and Kyle, both of whom are so understanding about the excessive demands of work and travel. Thanks to Mom, Dad, and my grandparents, who inspired in me not only a love of food, but a love of people, regardless of background. Our frequent family gatherings demonstrated time and time again how the simple act of sharing a meal can strengthen relationships, friendships, and connections.

Thanks are due to my longtime business partner, Doug Petkovic. You make me crazy most of the time, but I am forever grateful that you are always there for me in business, pleasure, and life in general as a true friend.

Thanks to Culinary Director Katie Pickens, whose painstaking recipe testing guarantees that every dish in this book will come out great. Over the past decade, Katie has become a member of the family. Corporate Chef Derek Clayton, my partner in crime, does all the heavy lifting to ensure that every plate in every restaurant is just as good (or better) as if I had made it myself. Here's hoping that one day, my friend, your glass will be half full!

Thanks to my manager of fifteen years, Scott Feldman of Two-Twelve Management, a real mensch who represents me as though I'm his only client. Nobody understands the food and media arena better than he does. Thanks also to Jon Rosen and William Morris Agency, a team that always manages to ink the perfect deal. Cheers to PR pro Becca Parrish, a longtime friend, and all her colleagues at BeccaPR, a team that always paints the perfect picture.

To my boy BFlay, a mentor who has grown to become a brother. You have helped me more than anyone to navigate the complex world of television while balancing the never-ending demands of restaurants and life.

This is the fifth book that I've collaborated on with Douglas Trattner, who not only is my coauthor, but is also a great and patient friend who puts up with my not-always-timely work assignments. For example, these acknowledgments that I am currently writing are due today! [Actually, these were due a month ago—Trattner]

Photographer Ed Anderson, along with Andie McMahon and Devon Grimes, has a knack for capturing the true spirit of the book while making every dish look as delicious on the page as it does in real life. It is always an honor and privilege to collaborate with super-stylist Susan Spungen, who brings another level of style, sophistication, and professionalism to everything she touches. This book is so much better because she was involved.

And, of course, Raquel Pelzel, our diligent and unflappable editor at Potter, who has kept this train on the tracks over the course of two books. She is always an absolute pleasure to work with.

Index